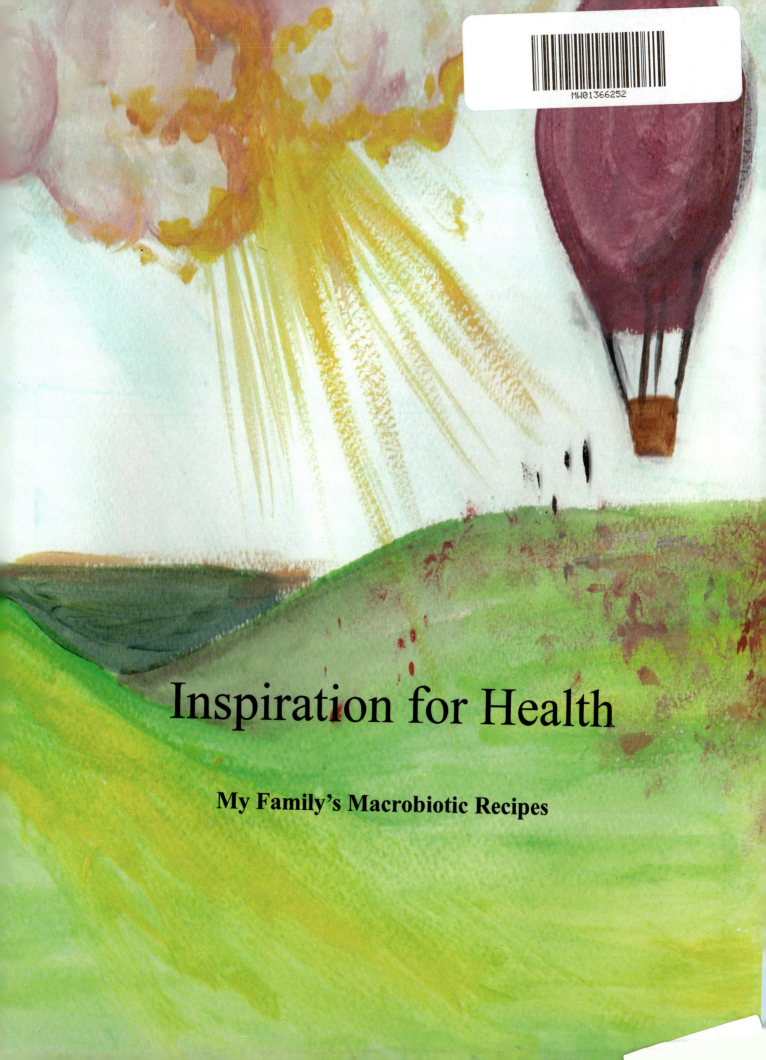

Inspiration for Health

My Family's Macrobiotic Recipes

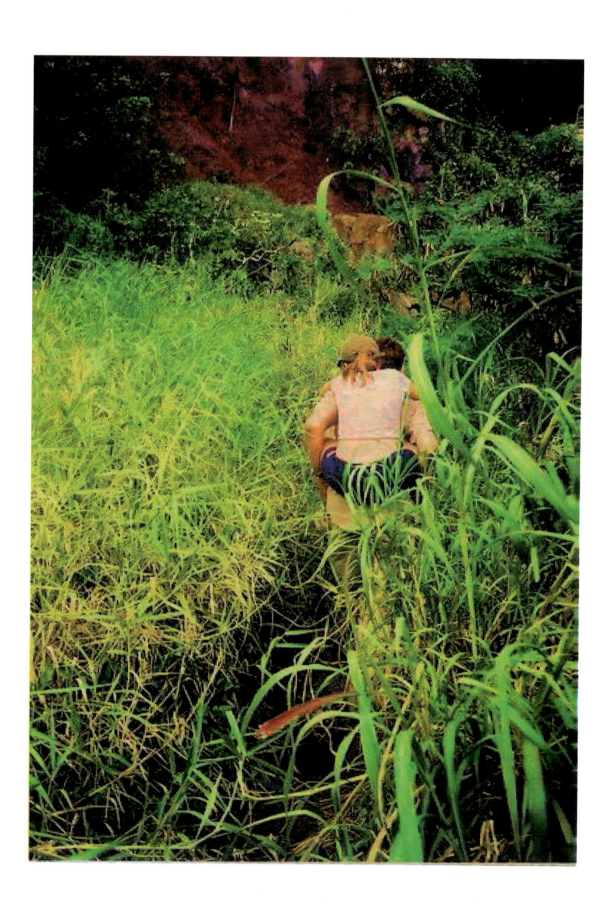

Published by ateasepress.com
All rights reserved including the right to reproduce this book, or parts thereof, in any form, except for the inclusion of brief quotations in a review.

At Ease Press
ISBN 978-0-917921-84-1
Copyright (c) 2008
Printed in the United States of America

For My Children
Alexander and Alicia

NOTICE

Inspiration for Health was originally written for my children, friends, family, and patients.
The recipes within this book are not intended as a substitute for treatments that are prescribed by your physician.

Acknowledgments

I look at life like a recipe.

It is my children, my friends and patients who are the ingredients of these recipes that make my life so fulfilling. **Inspiration for Healing** is dedicated to the ongoing love affair I have with my children and the patients I have had the privilege to work with over the last 25 years.

My children, Alexander and Alicia, I would to thank for all their support and patience. Being a single parent presented many challenges and scarifies for both my children and myself. Late nights, long nights, school plays I came late to and some I missed.

Thank you, *Baby Boy* and *Monkey Girl*.

I would also like to thank **Sister Margaret Antoine** who kept me in her prayers (and also edited this book in 2008).

My special love goes to the family of **Arthur Clokey** creator of **Gumby** who has supported **Inspiration for Health** and to my special friend **Joseph Pesci** whose kindness will always hold a special place in my heart. For **Father Peter Mary Rookey, Marge 1 and 2 and everyone at St. Michael's International Compassionate Ministry** *thank you* for the blessings, prayers, and inspirations to keep breathing.

My children, **Alex and Alicia** have been my support and my strength.

They are my reason in the morning and my prayer at the end of the day.

Through their eyes I see the world.

It is because of my children that I am who I am.

It is through their love that I hold to my faith and keep it every day.

I have kept with me for 40 years a **Happy Box** which holds my dreams and memories.

In my **Happy Box** is my daughter's poem called "**Wild Geese** "that she wrote in 2007.

I believe that her poem sums up everything

"Creation is the Healer for the soul

Friend for the lonely

Inspiration for the hopeless"

Special Thanks

Alicia and Alex
Alicia's best friend Teresa
Ana Fleming
Arthur Clokey
Susanne Handle
Daniel Marquex
Dan Brown
David Monier
Dr. George Ewing
Dr. Ron Carlson
Mark Arnett (father to my Harry P)
Elroy
George Moore
Harry Carmine
Jerimiah Gold
Jo Anne Walton
Joanne Tall
and
Joel
Kate
Mary
Roland Nip
Sea Gyspy Ladies
Stephanie Kimble
Steve and Turi
CPS for the State of Hawaii

And all my Patients

Inspiration for Health

My Family's Recipes

AA Austria

© 2008

My Family's Recipes are a collection of recipes that I have created for my own family and patients to assist in their health.The recipes are based on the **principles of macrobiotics** as well as an **Asian philosophy** of **healing through food**.

The traditional macrobiotic approach believes that **food and the quality of food** will directly affect an individual's health and well-being.

Macrobiotics emphasizes locally grown whole foods such as grains, vegetables, beans, fruits, nuts and seeds as well as various sea vegetables (kelp, wakame, dulse, hijiki, nori, arame, lavar, bladderwrack, and the various microalgaes   such as spirulina).

Brown rice and other whole grains such as barley, millet, oats, quinoa, spelt, rye, are incorporated in the planning of daily meals.

General guidelines are the following:

Whole cereal grains, especially brown rice: 40–60%

Vegetables: 25–30%

Beans / /legumes: 5–10%

Miso soups (barley, brown rice, soy) :   5%

Sea vegetables (kelp,wakame,dulse,hijakilavar,sea moss):   5%

Naturally processed foods (pickled daikon, mochi, spirulina) :   5–10%

Macrobiotic cooking follows the seasons.

In the spring and summer *lighter meals of steamed vegetables, fresh fruits and nuts and grains are emphasized.*

In the fall and winter *more concentrated foods are recommended such as pumpkin, stews, soups and heavier grains such as oats, spelt and kamut.*

Preservatives should be avoided as well as:

- Sugar
- Alcohol
- Honey
- Coffee
- Chocolate
- Refined flour products
- Very hot spices
- Recreational drugs

Food sources should be *pesticide and preservative free* and whenever possible *fresh* and *organic.*

Canned foods for purposes within this book should be *avoided* as well as *frozen, packaged and standard processed foods.*

Water should be *filtered* if the source is not trusted as well **as *chlorine* and *fluoride free.***

A gas stove is preferable over an electric.

Cookware should be stainless steel, glass or ceramic.

But above all

Cook with Love

Faith

and

Family

Appetizers

Alexander's Almond Sauce (1)

Black Macro Sesame Caviar (4)

Onion Macro Spread (7)

My Tofu Dill Sauce (10)

My Sweet Aspic (13)

Spinach Macro Flatbread (16)

Quesadillas and Jalapeno Hummus (19)

Goat Cheese Press (2

Salads

Alligator Pear Feta Salad (26)

Harry's Watercress Salad (29)

My Macro Waldorf Salad (32)

Soups

Alicia's Butternut Soup (35)

Black Bean Soup (38)

Carrot Beet Soup (41)

Creamy White Bean Slightly Spicy Soup (44)

Curried White Bean Soup (48)

French Curried Lentil Soup (51)

Soups

Kapiolani Tom Duc Soup (54)

Maderia Corn Chowder (57)

My French Onion Soup (60)

My Own Asparagus Soup (63)

My Own Papaya Soup (66)

LemonGrass Rice Noodle Soup (69)

Main Course

Alicia's Macadamia Nut Basil Pesto (72)

American Macro Artichoke Enchiladas (75)

American Macro Cornbread (79)

Artichokes with Goat Ricotta and Basil (82)

Feta Stuffed Bell Peppers (86)

Gingered Tofu Vegetables and Marian (90)

Golden Beets with Marinated Carrots (93)

Main Course

Grandma Evey's Long Bean and Rice (97)

Hand Held Nori (100)

Hallelujah Cashew (103)

Italian French Green Bean Sauté (108)

Hawaiian Macro Polenta (111)

Kathleen's Spicy Black Beans (114)

with Fiery Peppers

Main Course

Lotus Root Stuffed With Almond (119)

Louise's Stuffed Artichokes (123)

Macro Banana Squash with Wild Rice (125)

Macro Primavera Pasta Pie (128)

My Cabbage Roll Dumpling (132)

My Colorful Vegetable Casserole (136)

My Own Escarole Soup (139)

Main Course

Nana's Sugar Peas (142)

Popeyed Spinach Turnovers (145)

Sauté Almond French Long Beans (149)

Snuffy's Pea Pilaf (152)

Stuffed Kabocha Squash (155)

Stuffed Sweet Maui Onions (158)

Wok A Talk (161)

Desserts

American Macro Sweet Potato Pie (164)

Christmas Rice Pudding (167)

Holiday Kabocha Pumpkin Pie (170)

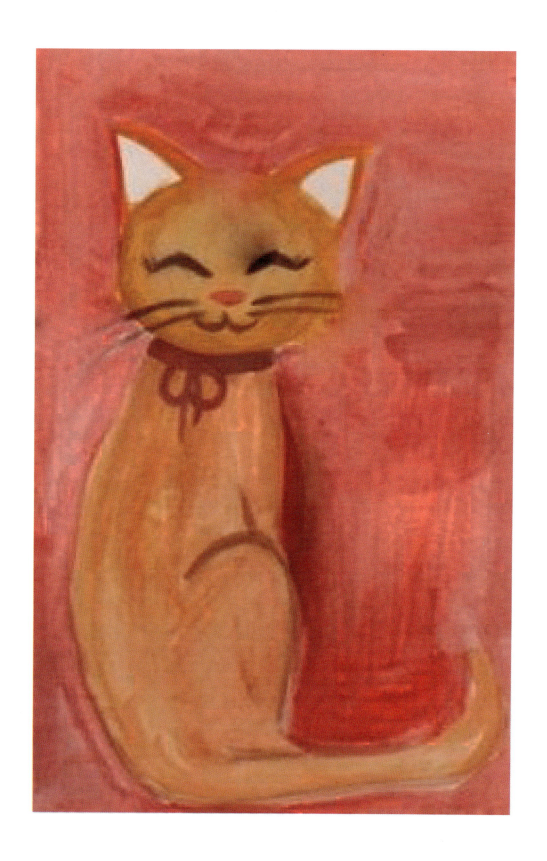

APPETIZER

Alexander's Almond Sauce

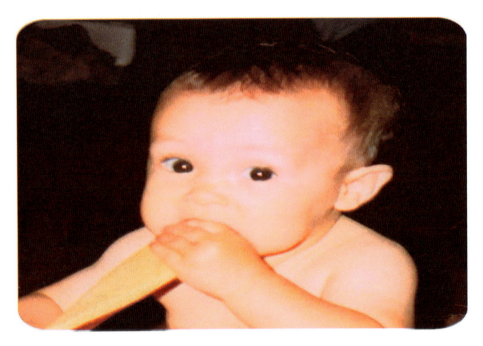

My son Alexander's favorite. **Alexander's Almond Sauce** *is my version of a Thai Peanut Satay. Thai kitchens in Hawaii traditionally use tamarind as a sweetener, crushed peanuts, coconut milk, garlic, and ginger with one or two stalks of fresh lemongrass in their satay recipe. Red saffron is gently folded into the mixture of peanuts and coconut milk then heated to enhance the flavor. Today, many Thai kitchens have surrendered to the easier and faster method of preparing their satay by using honey or brown sugar instead of tamarind, peanut butter instead of real peanuts, and extract of lemon for lemongrass. As many individuals have allergic reactions to peanuts,* **Alexander's Almond Sauce** *offers is a tasty alternative.*

Alexander's Almond Sauce

4 cups almond vanilla milk.
Masala or Thai curry red, yellow or green.
Red chili crushed.
Saffron to taste.
1 cup almonds, crushed.
¼ tsp. cumin powder.
¼ tsp. coriander powder.
1 tbsp. lemongrass or juice from 1 lemon/lime.
Raw honey, agave or brown rice syrup to taste

In a stainless steel pot:

Heat almond milk on low.
Slowly combine the remaining ingredients.
Simmer on very low for 30 minutes to one hour.
Stir frequently.
Serve over vegetables, noodles, rice and or tofu.

If desperate for a fast meal for the kids, prepared almond butter can be substituted in place of crushed almonds.
For the consistency you desire, simply add more almond milk or

Aruvadic medicine and Traditional Oriental Medicine often include almonds in many of their medicinal food recipes. Almonds are used to support the kidney/adrenal functions and are given a few at a time boiled, crushed or powdered to convalescing elderly within many Asian communities. Rich in protein, B and E vitamins, and the milk of the almond is a highly digestible food. Many dairy intolerant individuals will alternate almonds with other seed, grain or legume based milks. Sweet almonds are referred within the Bible as, **"among the best of fruit" (Genesis 43:11)**. *Chinese folklore regards the almond as* **"enduring sadness and female beauty"** *as the shape of the almond resembles a tear drop. Almonds have many uses. The almond nut can be made into milk, flour, and butter. Almond oil is an excellent skin moisturizer and the husks of the almond have commercial use as a building material. Almonds can also be made into soaps, used in shampoo, made into candies, prepared in cosmetics and used to exfoliate skin. In March of 2009 the Food and Drug Association in the United States recalled all peanuts in use as foods or commercially for their possible allergic reactions. It was at this time that almond prices rose worldwide*

Black Macro Sesame Caviar

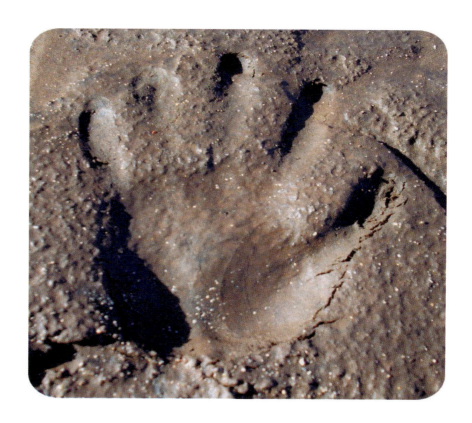

*I prepared this recipe for my family's Annual Thanksgiving Party in Cambria, California. Cambria is a community of retired individuals, artists and a vacation outlet. The friends and wonderful memories of my life there still hold a warm place in my heart. Especially memorable is the Thanksgiving Party I gave before to returning to Hawaii. Rows and rows of **Macro Foods** were devoured over two nights of celebration which included drumming, singing, laughing and eating. It was right after we lost the World Trade Center on 9/11. I have had many a Thanksgivings but none like the celebration on Thanksgiving Day 2003.*

Black Macro Sesame "Caviar"

1 cup black sesame seeds.
Olive oil.
Garlic powder to taste.

Grind sesame seeds into powder using food processor/coffee mill.
Mix oil, crushed sesame seed, garlic in a bowl.
Serve.

Can be eaten as a dip or spread.
Best served at room temperature.
Can be frozen for up to 38 days.

Rich in antioxidants and essential fatty acids, this caviar has traditional medicinal usages as an antifungal as well as an anti-parasitical. Black sesame seeds have been utilized in folk remedies for parasitical infections such as scabies where the oil of the seed is placed on the infection to smother the parasite. Chinese herbalists grind sesame seeds into a powder and taken as a tea to aide constipation. In Honolulu's Chinatown, during the Chinese New Year, sesame candies are given freely for good luck and good fortune for the coming year. Black sesame seeds have a type of plant phytoestrogen which is helpful during menopause. It is also helpful as a laxative and in reducing cholesterol. Sesame seeds are believed to have originated in India, and many variations can be found throughout China and East Asia. Sesame seeds when pressed produce an oil which is used in cooking or as a skin softener. The oil manufactured from the sesame seeds varies due to the type processing of the seed. Dark oil comes from the roasting of the sesame seeds, while lighter oil is usually from a cold press process.

Onion Macro Spread

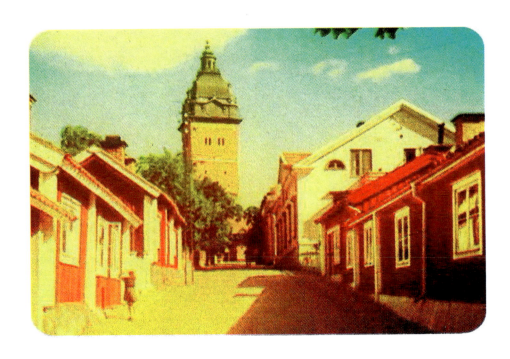

*I love all onions. I have a friend and longtime colleague, who in 1970 successfully walked from East Berlin into the West. One year when I was empty nesting as both my children had successfully entered into college. I realized that the holidays were upon us and it was Thanksgiving. I rented a cabin in Yosemite National Park in California with my two children Many of my friends gathered there to celebrate. We ate everything in sight and especially enjoyed the **Onion Macro Spread.** As we sat around the Franklin stove warming our hands and feet I noticed how over the years it is the company of close friends and warm memories that feed the heart and soul while my **Onion Macro Spread** feeds the spirit.*

Onion Macro Spread

1-2 red onions, peeled, washed, sliced.
1 cup fresh sweet basil.
1cup fresh parsley.
1tsp. kelp flakes.
1-3 tbsp. olive oil.
1 cup macadamia nuts, chopped.

In a stainless steel pot:

Steam onions to a soft consistency.
Puree nuts in blender / food processor until smooth.
Add steamed onions.
Puree all ingredients in a blender/ food processor.
Add olive oil, parsley, kelp flakes, basil.
Blend to a smooth consistency.
Serve hot over pasta, rice, or as a spread.

*The onion has throughout history been used for everything from curing a toothache to insect bites. The origin of the onion is not officially known, however one of the earliest recorded accounts **(Egyptian Book of the Dead)** gave reference to Egyptian folk medicine where the onion is given as a meal for infections. Europeans ate onions raw as well as cooked and made onions into syrup with raw honey as a cough medicine. Onions are found to be useful as an antimicrobial and antifungal in nature. When planted in a garden the odor from the onion can ward off pests and insects. Often times, individuals will experience a gastric complaint when eating onions (indigestion, hiccups, heartburn). These are transitory symptoms that can be eliminated or lessened by cooking onions. A tuber vegetable, onions can stay in the ground until harvested or stored in a dry area until needed. Onions can have a strong odor depending on the variety. Red sweet onions are relatively absent of odor when eaten raw or cooked, sweet yellow Bermuda onions are stronger in flavor and aroma while the white pearl onions can be eaten and cooked with little to no problem at all. Adding parsley when eating or cooking with onions will help eliminate odors.*

My Tofu Dill Sauce

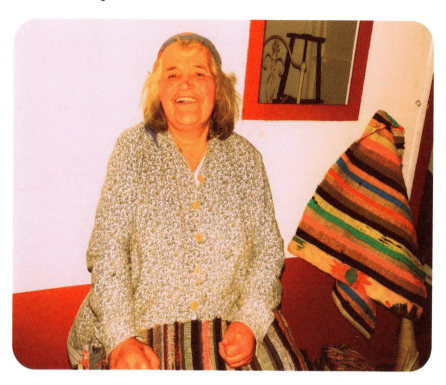

One of my patients was experiencing tremendous challenges with post menopausal symptoms. Hot flashes, night sweats, memory lost, weight gain and estreme fatigue that continued well after her menopause. After ten years of taradlitional hormone replacement therapy with very little positive effects, Danielle decided to "go natural". Her high blood pressure, diabetes and cholesterol were dramatically readuced through her lifestyle changes and embracing my macrobiotic program, and her post menopausal symptoms disappeared.

My Tofu Dill Sauce

1 lb. soft or silken tofu, cubed.
Juice of 1 lemon/lime.
Fresh or dry dill.

Blend tofu in food processor/blender until soft, creamy.
Fold in lemon and dill to taste.
Blend slowly.
Refrigerate overnight.
Serve.

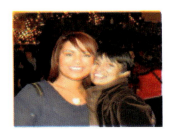

*High in plant estrogen, soy products provide a healthy alternative to traditional forms of hormone replacement therapy. In Asia, traditionally, women have had a lower incident of breast cancer in comparison to American or European women. The isoflavanoids found within soy products such tofu, tempeh, and fermented miso, have been studied and extensively researched regarding breast cancer. A study documented by the National Institute of Health in recently concluded after a ten year follow up with 35,308 Singapore women from 1993-1998 and then again in July of 2008 (**www.ncbI.nlm.nih.gov/pubmed/18594543**) that the intake of soy and its products reduced breast cancer risk in post-menopausal women of a leaner physical profile and recommended that 10mg. of soy for all postmenopausal women a day may have lasting beneficial effects against breast cancer development. There is some controversy over soy and soy products. As soy is a phytoestrogen individuals who do not benefit from estrogen products may want to limit or avoid consumption until condition improves as a precaution*

My Sweet Aspic

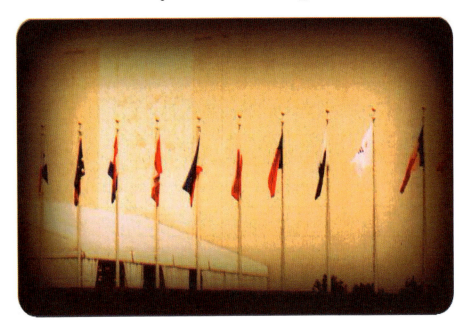

In 2003 in New York, I was requested to treat a Hungarian delegate to the United Nations. Her condition was a chronic gastrointestinal condition that had progressed over fifteen years. Medical treatment in Europe and the U.S. had proven to be ineffective. Within ten days, her condition improved and was reversed. Today, in her home in Budapest she is still following her nutritional program and incorporating it within her family. As a delegate to the United Nations with her heavy schedule both at the embassy and at home, her "healthy eating habits" is reflective within herself and the perfect health of her three children. **Sweet Aspic** *was specifically created for her while in New York for late night conferences at the U.N.*

My Sweet Aspic

2-4 cups yam, sweet potato, washed peeled and quartered.
1 cup carrots, sliced.
2 cups water.
1-2 tbsp. white miso.
Juice of 1 lemon/lime.
1 tbsp. arrowroot powder.
2-3 tbsp. black sesame seeds, roasted.
Lemon slices.
Parsley

In a stainless steel pot:

Boil water.
Combine vegetables with arrowroot.
Reduce heat to low.
Simmer for 10-15 minutes until all vegetables are soft and arrowroot is dissolved.
Stir often.
Remove from heat.
Dissolve miso in small amount of warm water in a cup.
Combine miso with mixture.
Simmer for 3-5 minutes.
Remove from heat.
Stir in lemon/lime juice.
Puree all ingredients in a blender/ food processor.
Pour into a cool casserole dish.
Let stand 30 minutes.
Refrigerate for 1-3 hours until solid and maintains form.
Cut into squares.
Serve and garnished with toasted black sesame seeds/or parsley.

*This recipe is useful for women who are entering menopause as well as for those who are depleted physically. "Yams" cause much confusion in the American market place. True "yams" are native to parts of Africa and Asia (**Discoreaceae family**) and have a traditional usage for hormonal support in African and Asian folk medicine. The "yam" is often confused with the "sweet potato". The appearance of the yam slightly differs from the sweet potato in that yams have a rougher skin and are darker in color with the meat ranging from orange to purple though some species can be white. In 1982, I studied with a brilliant gynecologist from Macau, Dr. Hok Chi Tsu, whose use of yams was incorporated in many herbal formulas. Traditionally, around the ages of 40 to 50 a **"yam cake"** was prepared for pre-menopausal women. Yams can be steamed, baked, boiled, mashed, made into a tea or used as a flour. Yams and sweet potatoes are very concentrated in beta-carotene an anti-oxidant which is necessary for skin repair. Cosmetics often use beta-carotene for treatment with wrinkles, sun damage and skin tone.*

Spinach Macro Flatbread

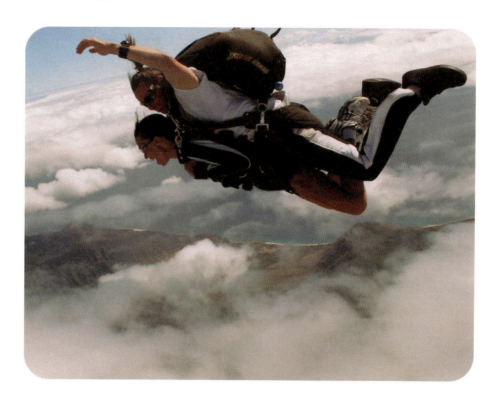

In 1993 I was diagnosed with Hashimoto's Thyroiditis after being exposed to pesticides from a Caltran truck in Northern California. My symptoms were extreme fatigue, palpitations, night sweats, hair and rapid weight loss. <u skin burned constantly, while the bottom of my feet peeled. Diagnosed with an autoimmune condition I was offered symptomatic treatment of point radiataion,surgical removal and medication for the thyroid. By 1995, my return to a traditional lifestyle with traditional medicianal support, enabled me to heal and to share my good fortune with others.

Spinach Macro Flatbread

1 wheat free/ yeast free flatbread (tortillas, laver, Armenian toast.).
5 tbsp. olive oil.
8 shallots, minced.
1 lb. fresh spinach, washed, dried with a paper towel
1 tsp. cayenne pepper.
1 cups carrots, shredded.
1 cup goat cheese feta, crumbled.
Kelp flakes.

Preheat oven to 375 degrees.

Heat bread on a baking sheet for 10 minute.
In a stainless steel skillet on low heat.

Heat oil and shallots.
Cook for 5 minutes.
Stir in spinach, cayenne pepper.
Remove from heat.

Transfer spinach, shallots, cayenne to large bowl.

Stir feta cheese into spinach mixture.
Spread spinach mixture onto bread.
Sprinkle evenly with shredded carrots.
Bake for 5-10 minutes, until bread begins to brown and cheese is melted.
Broil until golden brown.
Remove from oven
Slice and Serve.

*High in the nutrients zeaxanthin and lutein as well as other minerals and vitamins, spinach is noted to be very beneficial for vision. Though best eaten raw, the difficulty is the content of oxalic acid which inhibits iron absorption as well as calcium. Often symptoms of this inhibited function experienced as constipation. To help break down the iron content in spinach and circumvent the possible side effects, lemon or lime should be squeezed onto the spinach when eaten. Quickly boiling or lightly steaming spinach makes spinach easier to digest. Another reason for spinach's conspicuous avoidance is the odor that spinach produces when cooked. This is due mainly to the concentration of chlorophyll within its leaves and when heated omits a most unflavored smell. This may be one of the reasons that spinach is remarked as being the **number food that children all over the world dislike.***

Quesadillas and Jalapeno Hummus

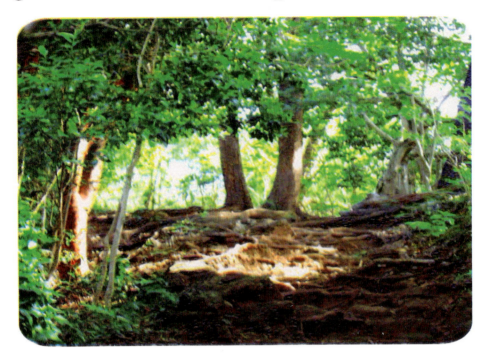

When both my children were young I had difficulty getting them to eat anything. Their childhood memories of corn and rice tortillas with goat cheese, rice and vegetables eaten as children became their comfort food as adults. Once, when the power had gone out from strong winds thirteen pine trees had fallen across our property. I found my children wrapped in a sleeping bag on my bed, asleep with their cold quesadillas beside them. When I asked my children why they didn't go to the neighbors, their answer was that "they did not want me to come home and eat alone". This recipe is for all the working single parents and the great kids who never let us eat alone.

Quesadillas and Jalapeno Hummus

Olive oil.
1 lb. extra firm tofu, cubed.
1 scallion, sliced.
1 tbsp. macadamia nuts, chopped.
1 carrot, shredded.
1 jalapeno, de seeded, chopped.
8 rice/ spelt flour tortillas.
1 cup sheep/goat Monterey jack, shredded.
Hummus (see recipe below).

Preheat oven to 350 degrees
In a stainless steel skillet:

Sauté tofu, onion in oil.
Place sauté tofu, onion in bowl.
Set aside.

Add nuts to skillet.
Stir nuts until golden.
Remove from skillet and heat.

In an oven safe casserole dish:

Place 4 tortillas on the bottom.
Spread a generous amount of hummus on each tortilla.
Top with tofu and scallions...
Then cheese and nuts.
Sprinkle with carrots.
Place 4 tortillas on top of the previous layer.
Repeat tofu, cheese, nuts, cilantro, and carrots mixture until all tortillas are gone.

Place in oven.

Bake until cheese is melted.
Remove from heat.
Slightly cool.
Cut into wedges.
Serve.

Hummus:

1 cup garbanzo beans.
6-8 cloves garlic, minced.
1 jalapeno, chopped.
Juice of one lemon.
Parsley.
Olive oil.

Soak beans overnight.
Drain.

In a stainless steel pot:

Cover beans with water.
Cook on low until soft.
Place all ingredients in blender/ food processor.
Blend until smooth.
Add in jalapeno.
Serve with quesadilla.

*Garbanzo or "chick peas" as they are also known as, are large bumpy legumes that resemble peas. Popular in middle eastern foods and a staple in India, chick peas have been cultivated for over 10,000 years. A cold weather crop, chick peas are harvested at the end of winter. Very susceptible to a variety of vegetable blights, chick pea cultivation takes skill in safe chick pea production. Varieties of the chick pea are found throughout the world ranging from the Middle East to South America to the Philippines. Mature fresh chick peas are often ground into flour and used in many forms as an alcoholic beverage, or to make an East Indian meat substitute (**falafel**). Chick peas can be dried, sprouted or eaten fresh. Very nutritious, the chick pea is a good source for vegetable protein as well as calcium. The chick pea is a food staple in the Middle East and eaten in the form of "**hummus**" and in the traditional falafel the "**sandwich**" of Egypt. A very digestible legume which is made easier for the body to assimilate when including lemon or lime juice to the recipes.*

Goat Cheese Press

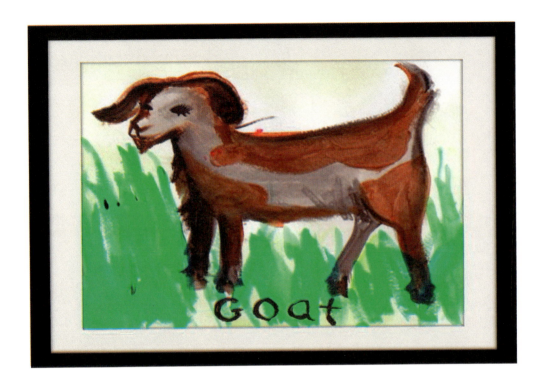

Goat milk *is often used as a substitute with dairy intolerant individuals. Goat and sheep products have traditionally been used to increase lactation for birth mothers. Strong in flavor, goat and sheep products often produce less allergenic reactions in comparison to dairy products. This may be due primarily to a less offensive form of lactose within the goat milk. With this recipe, I use lots of minced fresh garlic mixed with the cheese age for weeks in the freezer. Sheep and goat milk production usually occurs in spring time and declines at the end of fall. Today goat and sheep products are available year round.*

Goat Cheese Press

1 lb. goat/sheep cream cheese.
1 cup macadamia nuts.
Fresh or dry rosemary.
Garlic, minced.
1-1 ½ cup olive oil.

In a bowl:

Mix all ingredients...
Freeze until needed.
Serve on wheat free toast, use as a dip or mix with warm vegetables.

During the Christmas holidays, I substitute fresh figs or unsultured cranberries for olive oil and garlic for a festive flavor.

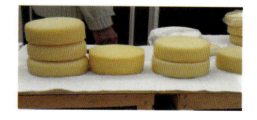

*There are many species of goats. Nubian goats are known for their milk products. Cashmere goats are prized for their beautiful long hair which is made into cashmere wool. Milk goats are the "nannies" while a male goat is used for his meat and is known as a "buck" or "Billy". Young goats are referred to as "kids". Goats are mentioned in Norse mythology (Thor's chariot was pulled by goats), the zodiac (**Capricorn**), and throughout the Old and New Testament in the Bible (**Exodus25:4, Matthew 25**). Very intelligent and curious, goats make excellent pets as they are easily trained and protective. Goat products are as versatile as dairy products and are quickly replacing dairy as an alternative in foods and in commercial production. Environmentally, goats are more effective as a reliable food source as goats are less toxic in nature. The gas "methane" has become an issue and concern worldwide. Extremely toxic, methane is produced as a byproduct from the fecal matter of cattle. Cattle production remains constant in its methane production. Sheep and goat production are economically and environmentally being reviewed as a viable alternative today worldwide.*

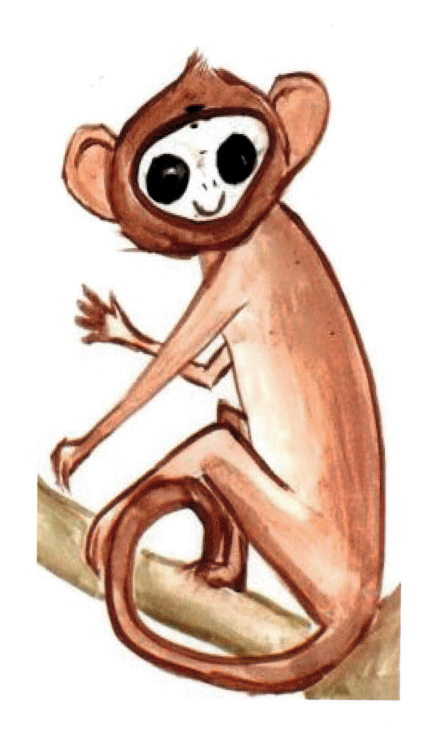

SALADS

Alligator Pear Feta Salad

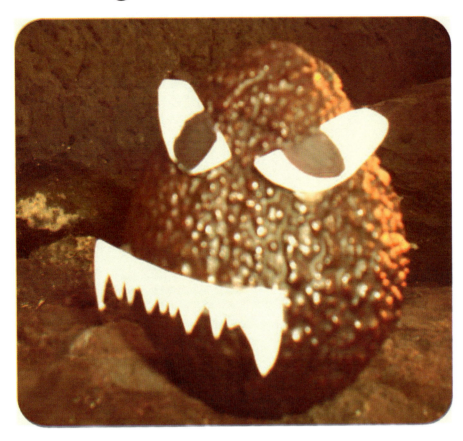

When I was young I was afraid of the color green. My family tried to encourage me to eat new foods and the avocado was one of them. They even tried to disguise the avocado. As a youngster, the avocado looked like an alligator that was shaped like a pear. This is how I refer to the avocado still to this day. I have used different styles of pasta for this recipe as well as different varieties of lettuce greens. I prefer the penne pasta for this recipe, althoughmy daughter prefers the rigatoni. As for my fear of the avocado, well somedays…

Alligator Pear Feta Salad

Wheat free penne or other styles of pasta.
Red romaine, arugula, oak or butter lettuce.
½ cup olive oil.
¾ cup carrots, shredded.
½ cup goat/sheep feta, crumbled.
½ cup scallions thinly sliced.
½ cup black olives, chopped.
3 tbsp. parsley, chopped.
1 garlic clove, minced.
2 avocados, skins peeled off.
Macadamia nuts, chopped.
1 tbsp. lemon juice.

In stainless steel pot:

Cook pasta, al dente.
Drain.
Place pasta in a bowl.
Toss with olive oil/garlic.
Fold in carrots, feta, onions, parsley, and minced garlic.
Chill.
Mix with lettuces.
Bring salad to room temperature before serving.
Cut avocados into cubes.
Toss with lemon juice.
Fold avocado into salad.
Sprinkle with toasted macadamia nuts.
Serve.

The avocado was first discovered by Spanish conquistadors in Mexico and eventually brought over to Europe and North America. At first the avocado was viewed as a tasteless food that most individuals would shy away from. The avocado is classified as a "fruit' and was viewed as one of the most unpopular fruits until the mid-1960. The avocado's popularity increased as a result of cultural regional diversity that became worldwide due to integration of ethnicity through media. Television increased the awareness in differences and similarities within cultures by introducing many culturally traditional foods. **Guacamole***, an avocado paste mixed with cilantro, tomatillos, red pepper and lime became the appetizer on everyone's menu. Aztec Indians ate avocados as an aphrodisiac and rubbed the meat of the avocado on their skin to protect them from the sun and also as a moisturizer. Avocados are high in Vitamin E, Vitamin C and have more potassium than bananas. Also avocados are low in calories and contain unsaturated oils that are beneficial in maintaining good cholesterol.*

Harry's Watercress Salad

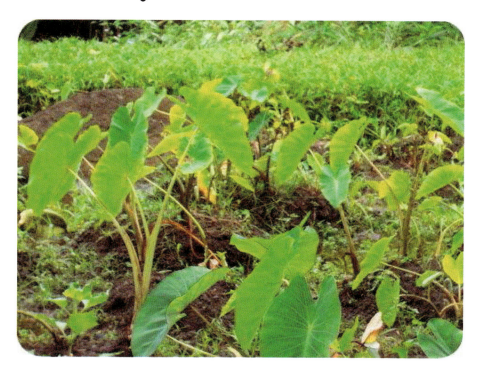

*While living onMaui, I worked in the poi patches near Hana with my adopeted Uncle Harry. Uncle had me standing in water and mud all day long pulling what I then thought was weeds. Years later I realized it was watercress and I can still hear Uncle saying to me, "**You know, you can always eat it**". Harry was a **kahuna lapalahau**, an herbalist who was practiced in the tradition of oral folk history, known as "talk story". Hawaiian language until recently was all but forgotten and not at all spoken except by a few and mainly on the outer islands .The **Ohana** (family) movement with Uncle Harry and others , have returned the traditions and dignity of Hawaii for our **keiki** (young) and for the world.*

Harry's Watercress Salad

1 lb. asparagus, ends removed.
1 lb. watercress, cleaned.
8 oz. hard goat cheese, graded.
1 cup almonds, crushed.
1 tbsp. cilantro, chopped.
3 tbsp. olive oil.
1 lemon or lime.

In a stainless steel pot with a steamer basket:

Steam asparagus.
Mix watercress with cilantro.
Arrange watercress on a serving dish.
Place asparagus on top of watercress.
Top with cheese, almonds.
Mix olive oil with lemon/ lime.
Sprinkle on watercress.
Serve.

*Watercress is a semi aquatic plant that originated in Europe. It grows year round and is one of the oldest leaf vegetables consumed (**Wikipedia**) by humans globally. Botanically, watercress resides in the family of mustard which attributes to its bitter peppery flavor. Unstable as a dry herb, watercress is best eaten fresh. It is useful as a diuretic and high in Vitamin C. Traditional uses of watercress have been as a tonic, for breathing conditions, colds, flues, and more. Poultices have been applied for cuts, boils and rashes. Beneficial as an agent in the production of bile in the body, watercress has the reputation for detoxification of the body. Many believe that the watercress is beneficial for vision as the abundance of magnesium maintains muscle strength and integrity thereby allowing ocular muscles to help maintain ocular efficacy. Hawaii is unique in its variety of watercress that is grown locally on Oahu, Maui and the Big Island. This local watercress has long green stalks and large leaves that make it desirable year round and one of Hawaii's most desirable salad greens on any tale.*

My Macro Waldorf Salad

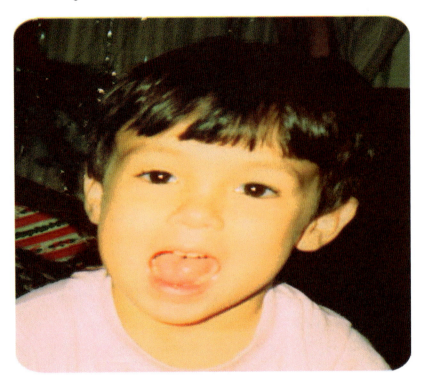

*When my children were young, salads were an ordeal. Sunday brunch at the Wisteria restaurant in Honolulu was usually the only time my children had what we called **"mainland lettuce"**. In Hawaii, the lettuce that many of us are familiar with, is **Ogo**, a local kelp. Not too long ago I remember picking fresh ogo along many Hawaiian shorelines. Today, sewer pipes from the overflow of housing make many of our local sea foods dangerous and toxic. **My Macro Waldorf Salad** minus the walnuts and iceberg lettuce is for my children in memory of Sundays at the Wisteria.*

My Macro Waldorf Salad

Dressing:

¼ cup olive oil.
¼ cup lemon/lime juice.
1 tbsp. dark toasted sesame oil.
1 tbsp. Braggs Liquid Amino Acids.
¼ tsp. fresh ginger, grated.
Freshly ground black pepper to taste.

Place all ingredients in blender or food processor.
Blend until smooth.
Set aside.

Salad:

1 head butter leaf or red leaf romaine.
1 cup wakame, shredded.
3 cups cauliflower.
¼ cup carrot, shredded.
¼ cup zucchini, shredded.
Peeled and cubed apples.
¼ cup raw macadamia nuts, crushed.

In a large bowl:

Toss lettuce, cauliflower, carrot, macadamia nuts,apples and zucchini.
Drizzle dressing over salad.
Toss.
Spoon salad onto serving plate.
Sprinkle crushed macadamia nuts over salad.

*The red romaine lettuce is a warm weather crop that medicinally has been used in folk medicine for insomnia, constipation and as a diuretic. Originally, lettuce was cultivated by the Greeks and Romans as an aphrodisiac. Romaine lettuce is bitter in flavor and comparatively stronger in taste than the familiar iceberg lettuce. Similar in taste and usage to the red romaine, are the red and green oak leaf lettuce. The original Waldorf Salad was created for the opening of the Waldorf Hotel in New York in 1893 which eventually became the Waldorf Astoria Hotel. The original recipe was very simple and included apples, celery, walnuts and an egg based mayonnaise. My version of the Waldorf Salad is worlds apart from **Oscar Tschirky** (creator of the Waldorf salad) recipe. The addition of **wakame** (a sea vegetable) compliments the romaine lettuce and boosts the metabolism. I include Hawaiian macadamia nuts in place of walnuts to assist in cholesterol reduction. Also, apples are absent from my recipe as I believe the combination of fruits with vegetables can create difficulty in the body's ability to process and assimilate necessary nutrients.*

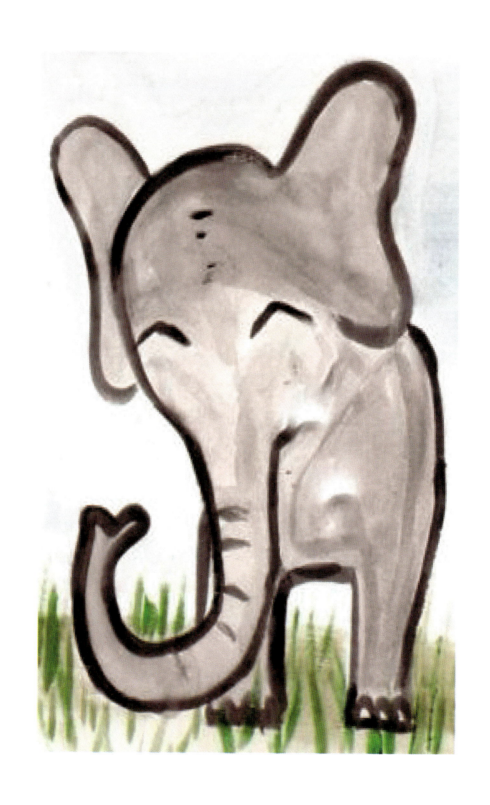

SOUP

ALICIA'S BUTTERNUT SOUP

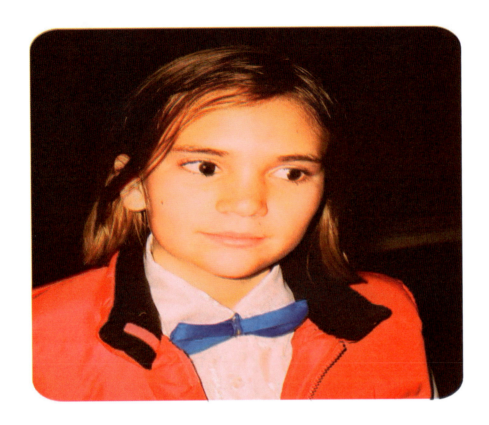

At nine years old, my daughter had already decided what she would and would not eat. When cooking for my daughter, color, smells, taste, had to be taken into careful consideration. Too thick, too thin, too hot, too cold; it was as if I was feeding Goldilocks every day. Finally, this version of **Butternut Soup** *was so satisfying that Alicia would eat a whole bowl without any coaching, begging or goldfish crackers.* **Alicia's Butternut Soup** *is sweet and light, just like my girl. Also,* **Alicia's Butternut Soup** *has the* **children's stamp of approval**

ALICIA'S BUTTERNUT SOUP

1 butternut squash, washed, quartered, and de-seeded.
1 lb. carrots, sliced.
1 leek or green onions, sliced.
1 garlic bulb, minced.
1-2 tsp. white miso.
Tarragon, sweet basil, chervil to taste.
Rice, almond, soy, multigrain, or oat milk.
Sheep/goat Pecorino Romano, grated.
Cinnamon.

Place in a stainless steel pot with a steamer basket.

Steam all the vegetables together.
Remove from heat.
Remove vegetables from pot.
Place vegetables in blender/food processor.
Add one cup of liquid from steaming the vegetables.
Blend to liquid consistency.

In stainless steel pot:

Place blended vegetables.
Mix in miso.
Add milk to desired thickness.
Add spices.
Simmer for 30 minutes on low.
Serve with goat/sheep pecorino or nondairy sour cream.
Top with cinnamon.

*The butternut squash is a gourd that grows on a vine on the ground. It is believed to have originated from Mexico and has many medicinal usages. The seeds are valued highly for their anti-parasitical properties. The meat of the butternut can be steamed, mashed or made into a liquid which enables an easier digestion for convalescing individuals. The butternut squash is abundant in antioxidants, minerals, and vitamins, particularly Vitamin A. When dried, the rind of the butternut has been used as an ornament, a musical instrument, to preserve liquids, and in religious ceremonial practices. The size of the butternut can vary from 6 inches in length to 2 feet or larger. For some though, the rind of the butternut squash can produce a contact dermatitis resulting in red itchy skin. Traditional oriental medicinal use of the butternut squash taken in food formulas is used for treating bouts of depression, insomnia and anxiety. The butternut squash is very easy to digest and assimilate. It is beneficial for digestive disorders as Vitamin A and its pro vitamin A, **beta-carotene**, is essential in tissue repair.*

Black Bean Soup

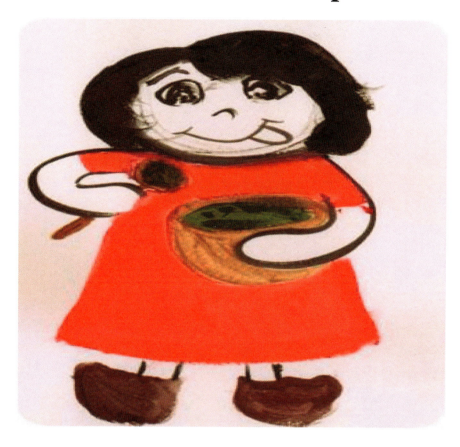

*I should call this "**David's Soup**". He reminds me that this is his favorite, although he is quick to add, "That everything you cook is my favorite". This is my version of a Creole classic prepared on **"Laundry Day Mondays"**. **Black Bean Soup** was traditionally made in large pots slowed cooked all day long in outside kitchens. David adds extra red peppers, cayenne and saffron to the black beans just enough, he says, " **to make the sidewalks steam**". I often wondered with so much "heat "in the soup, would it also help the laundry dry faster.*

Black Bean Soup

1 4-6inch kelp washed and rinsed.
2-3 cups black beans, washed and rinsed.
1 leek or 1 red onion, sliced.
Red pepper, chili pepper, tarragon, sweet basil to taste.
1-2 tbsp. white miso to taste.

In a crock pot:

Place kelp on bottom.

Combine remaining ingredients in crock pot.
Cover with water.
Cook on low over night.
Season to taste.
Serve.

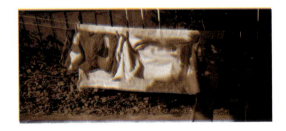

Black beans are high in protein, but are often difficult to digest. Soaking over night or slow cooking reduces the fibrous quality of the black beans while the addition of kelp softens the hard outer shell of the beans. Native to South America, black beans are a warm weather crop. Grown on vines black beans require a dry climate to flourish and an abundance of water. In traditional oriental medicine the color black is associated with the function of the kidneys and adrenals. This may be why traditional oriental practitioners incorporate black beans in many food formulas to enrich the body's kidney and adrenal system incorporating the beans to act as a tonic. Dried, soaked,, sprouted, made into a flour, added to soups , prepared as a paste, and made into candies are just a few of the many uses for this **Frijoles Negros.** *In the Chinese New Year black bean cakes are given as special pastries during the 1 month celebration to ensure a healthy body for the coming year.*

Carrot Beet Soup

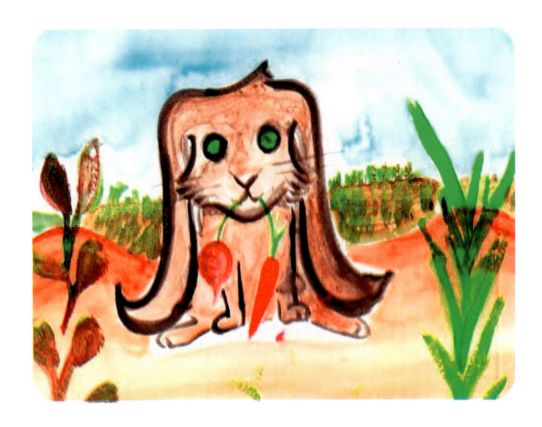

*Traditionally, the beet had been used for many of women's hormonal challenges. Conditions such as cysts, fibroids, menopausal and fertility problems have long employed beets into the diet. The beet can have a strong taste for many so the addition of carrots sweetens the flavor. Many of my patients prefer simply blending this recipe as a sort of **juicing experience**, though I prefer the **slow cooking** approach. Enjoying **Carrot Beet Soup** either as a "**juice** or as a "**soup**" is a matter of individual preference. When asked which form of **Carrot Beat Soup** did my patients prefer, juice or soup, they will simply reply, "**Both**".*

Carrot Beet Soup

1 red beet, cleaned sliced, quartered.
1 leek or red onion, peeled, washed, chopped.
6 carrots, sliced.
6 garlic cloves, minced
1-2 tsp. each basil, sweet tarragon to taste.
1 tbsp. lemon/lime juice.
1-2 tbsp. light miso.
6 cups of water.

In a stainless steel skillet:

Sauté leek/green onions, garlic.

In stainless steel pot:

Simmer vegetables in 6 cups of water until soft.
Add garlic and onions.
Puree veggies in blender/ food processor.

Return to pot

In a cup of warm water add miso.
Stir until dissolved.
Add miso and lemon/lime to puree.
Simmer 5-10 minutes.
Add water if needed.
Serve

Beets contain a high level of soluble and insoluble fiber. Traditional oriental practitioners have employed beets in women's health for the treatment of uterine fibroids, hot flashes, endometriosis and menstrual disorders. Beets are also high in carotenoids and betaine, antioxidants that improve skin structure, strength and integrity. In traditional oriental medicine the beet is one of the signature vegetables for women's herbal medicine. The many varieties of beets are valued for their individual tastes and textures. Especially prized is the **Golden Beet** cultivated for its smooth body and light meat. When preparing beets it is advisable to wear kitchen gloves for protection from the very strong liquid that the beet produces. Also, covering the work space where the beet will be prepared is highly advisable. Similar to spinach and chard, beet leaves are bitter in taste and as they contain oxalic acid are difficult to digest and are best avoided if constipation is a challenge. Beets today are most notably known for their commercial use in sugar production in direct competition with the sugar cane and are cultivated mainly in China

Creamy White Navy Bean Slightly Spicy Soup

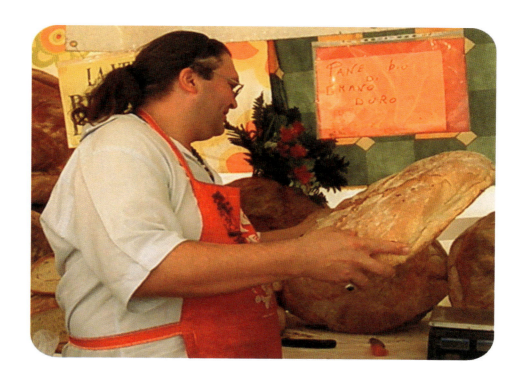

*My friend **"Hollywood Chef,"** introduced me to this small, smooth white bean, the star of this recipe, the cannellini. Personal chef to a family in the East Coast, we worked together preparing meals for each family member and writing their individual health programs. When everything was said and done, several programs were developed that Chef Hollywood could prepare and also that the family would eat. Often times, the chefs that I work with are "stand offish" at best, but this Hollywood chef was warm and caring and I can certainly appreciate why his East Coast family loves him so.*

Creamy White Navy Bean Slightly Spicy Soup

1 cup cannellini beans.
3-6 inch kelp, washed.
2-4 carrots, sliced.
1 leek or green onion, peeled, washed, sliced.
2-6 cloves garlic, minced.
4 cups almond milk.
1 tsp. tarragon.
Chili pepper, cayenne, red pepper to taste.
2-3 tbsp. olive oil (more if desired).

Place beans in crock pot.

Add kelp.
Soak overnight.
After soaking:
Drain fluid from beans.
Remove and discard kelp.

Set aside.

In a stainless steel skillet:

Sauté onions, fresh garlic, carrots until onions are a clear opaque color in olive oil.
Place with 2/3 of cooked beans in blender/ food processor.
Puree until smooth.

In a stainless steel pot

Combine carrots, garlic, onions to the bean mixture.
Add almond milk to bean mixture.
Simmer on low.

Stir.
Add milk to pot until desired thickness is obtained.
Add tarragon, garlic to pot.
Add 2 tbsp. of olive oil (more if desired) to pot.
Add peppers to taste.
Simmer on low for 1 hour.
Serve.

*Cannelloni beans are a white Italian kidney bean. Sometimes referred to as the "**Great Northern Bean**", the cannellini bean is made easier to digest if soaked overnight. If salt or any salt substitute is added it is advisable to add after cooking as the salt dries and toughens the outer skin of this bean. Cannellini beans are an excellent food choice for the iron, magnesium and B vitamins. As with many legumes, the cannellini bean is helpful w in diets for coronary heart disease, diabetes, and high cholesterol. Rich in protein, the benefits of this bean are recorded throughout history in many European folk remedies. Smooth and white in appearance, traditional practitioners of oriental medicine believe that this bean is helpful for the strengthening of the kidney and adrenals. When cooking with the cannellini bean, the addition of Kombu (kelp) further softens the fibrous makeup of the cannelloni bean as well as increasing minerals and vitamin content by breaking down the hard outer shell. As many legumes have a nitrous quality, soaking overnight and slow cooking either in a crock pot or on a gas range will help reduce this problem.*

Curried White Navy Bean Soup

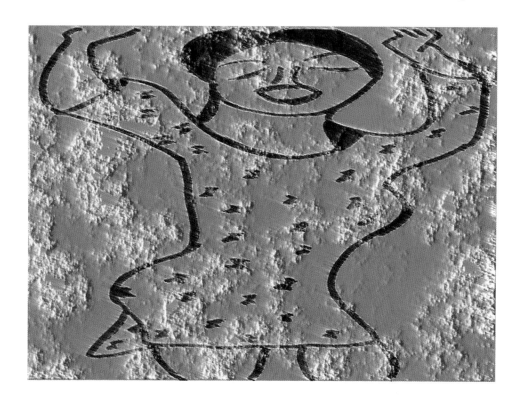

*My patients tell me that they love **Black Bean Cajun Style Soup** more than anything, however, my version of **Curried White Navy Bean Soup** comes in a close second as long as I keep it extra hot. Soaking the beans overnight helps to break down the hard shell of the legume as does slow cooking in a crock pot. Adding kelp further breaks down the tough fibrous texure of the bean while adding minerals and vitamins to the soup. My patients tell me that they prefer this soup a day or two later allowing the spices to simmer and create a stronger flavor. Who am I to argue.*

Curried White Navy Bean Soup

1-2 cups uncooked white navy bean, washed, drained.
1 3-6inches kelp, washed.
6-8 carrots, sliced.
1-2 leeks or green onion, washed, peeled, sliced.
1 cup julienne green beans or 1-2 zucchini, sliced.
1-3 tbsp. yellow, green or red curry.
1 garlic bulb, minced.
1-2 tbsp. ginger, grated.
1 tsp. each basil, cumin,cinnmon.
1-3 tbsp. olive oil.
4 cups almond milk.

In bottom of crock pot.

Place kelp.
Place beans, carrots, leeks/onions, green beans, zucchini, olive oil, herbs, and spices in crock pot.
Fill crock pot with water to cover beans and vegetables.
Slow cook on low over night.
As water cooks down add milk and seasoning.
Simmer on low for 30 minutes or longer to desired consistency.
Serve

Curry is a spice that has been used in many parts of the world, especially India. Until recently, many locations in India did not have suitable refrigeration or proper food storage. Curry acts as a natural preservative keeping the quality of the food in a stable condition for longer periods of time. Depending on the temperature of the curry will determine the use of this recipe. The hotter the curry, the more warming the soup. The milder the curry, the more nurturing this recipe becomes. Curry also helps in breaking down the outer shell of the white beans aiding digestion and assimilation of the minerals, vitamins and proteins. Curry's versatility in taste and flavor are reflected across continents in color and preparations. Whether the curry is a Masala or a Tamil. From India or Japan, red, yellow or green, curry adds a flavor that is distinctive for each meal. Curry can be added in soups, combined with rice and vegetables, added as an ingredient in chocolate or prepared as a beverage. In India, curry is also used as dye for clothing. In parts of Africa, curry is used ceremonially to color the skin in rites of passage for boys as well as for girls.

FRENCH CURRIED LENTIL SOUP

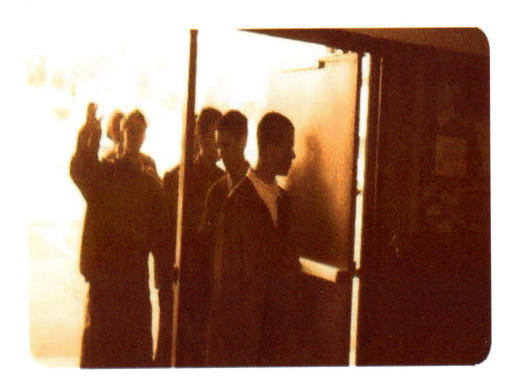

Compared to other street drugs, methamphetamine is at first relatively inexpensive ranging in price from $30 a gram to $300. In interviewing teenagers, many of their first introduction to "Ice", was to lose weight. Meth is a "cheap man's" cocaine and highly addictive. Dealers will target youngsters in parks, schoolyards, or beaches. At first giving the drugs for free, then in time using the children to become carriers or "mules" for the dealers. Hawaii is #1 for chrystal meth addition in the U.S. today. To assist in the epidemic, **Habilitat,** *based in Hawaii, provides a long term in house residential rehabilitation program to help with substance abuse.*

French Curried Lentil Soup

1 lb. French lentils, washed, rinsed.
1 5 inch kelp, washed.
4-6 carrots, sliced.
1 leek or red onion, peeled, washed, sliced.
1 garlic bulb, minced.
1-2 tbsp. masala curry or green Thai curry.
2-3 tbsp. olive oil.
Crushed chili pepper to taste.
Juice of one fresh lemon.
Fresh or dry dill to taste.
1 cup almonds, crushed.
Lemongrass or 1 lemon, sliced.
Sheep/goat Romano pecorino, grated.

In a crock pot:

Place kelp at bottom.
Add lentils, carrots, leeks or onions.
Add lemon/lemongrass and almonds.
Cover with water.
Slow cook on low in crock pot over night.
Add spices, herbs to taste.
As water cooks down after overnight,
Add rice or almond milk to desired consistency.
Remove lemon/lemongrass and discard.
Sprinkle cheese, almonds as desired on lentils.
Serve

The French lentil is very high in vegetable protein and is one of the most utilized protein sources the world. Originating between East Asia and the Mediterranean coast, lentils are a staple in many countries where vegetarian diets are common. The French lentil is comparably smaller than the common green lentil and far more delicate. It is also lighter in taste and texture. Many chefs prefer using the French lentil in their cooking. Slow cooking or overnight soaking softens the lentils, breaking down its outer shell. The addition of kelp further aides in breaking down the legumes while adding minerals and vitamins to the soup. In Jewish folk medicine, it is believed that the lentil is shaped like a tear and given during times of grief and grieving. It is an eternal symbol for birth, life and death. As a legume, the lentil's shell is comparatively softer than many of the other beans and requires a shorter cooking time. In India, the lentil is known as "dhal" and can be a light orange, bright red or yellow. I use this soup to nurture the body with its easy assimilation of protein for individuals who are physically depleted as well as to nourish the spirit. ..

KAPIOLANI TOM DUC SOUP

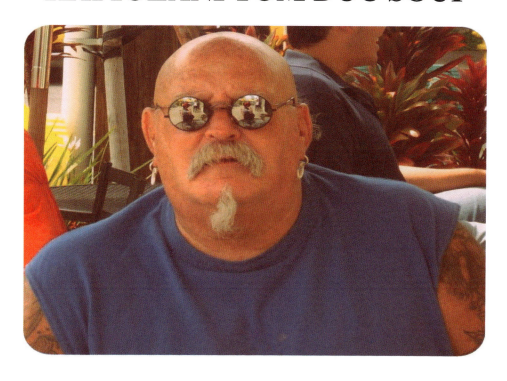

In 1995 I started the Kapiolani Homeless Shelter in Honolulu, Hawaii. It was there that I met and treated Fred Pepper, a decorated Vietnam Veteran suffering from PTSD, Post Traumatic Stress Disorder. In 2009, cases of PTSD in solders returning from Afghanistan were triple the amount recorded from any previous war in the United States . Fred has been noted in many publications for his contributions for the Veterans of the Vietnam War and his assistance with their surviving dependents. Often seen in Honolulu riding his Harley with a teddy bear tied to the rear seat, Fred continues to assist and serve. Well loved by all and especially by my family.

KAPIOLANI TOM DUC SOUP

4 cups vanilla almond milk or other nondairy milk.
4-6 carrots, sliced.
1 leek or 1 green onion, sliced.
2 zucchini sliced in half moons and quartered.
4-6 leaves of bok Choy, sliced.
Thai green curry for mild taste/ red curry for a stronger flavor.
2 tbsp. olive oil.
Rice noodles, or brown rice.

In a stainless steel pot:

Place carrots, zucchini in almond milk.
Simmer on very low so as not to curdle milk.
Add spices to milk.

In a stainless steel skillet:

Sauté leeks/ onions and bok Choy in olive oil.
Add leeks/onions, bok choy to ingredients in pot.
Simmer low for 30 minutes to one hour or longer.
Stir often.
Serve over rice or bean thread rice noodles.

Traditional Oriental Practitioners believe that the body's ability to digest and assimilate nutrients from foods is what maintains and restores health. Plant or grain based milk provide easily digestible proteins. When combined with the ingredients in this recipe, a complete nutritional profile of protein, vitamins and minerals help rebuild and restore the health of an individual. This formula is effective when individuals are convalescing both physically and emotionally. Post-Traumatic Stress Disorder (PTSD) is a physical and emotional condition that develops after exposure to a traumatic event (www.nih.gov/healthtopicstress). Positive involvement with family, friends and their environment is paramount for individuals with PTSD in learning trust, building confidence and regaining a fulfilling live. Individuals with PTSD report feeing ambiguous to their surroundings, distant from loved ones often reliving their trauma in dreams, memories and daily lives. PTSD occurs as a direct result from assaults, disasters, accidents and military combat. Treatment through various therapies can help control an overcome eventually PTSD.

Madera Corn Chowder Soup

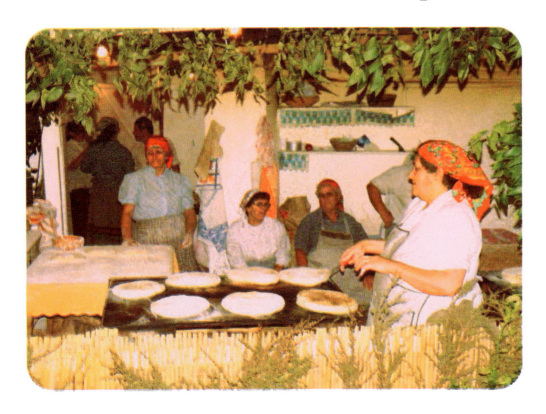

This recipe is a variation of the Mexican classic, **"Corn Tortilla Soup"** *without the tortillas (you can add a corn tortilla if desired). While traveling in Portugal I met women who prepared meals on outside stoves. Their "tortillas" were thick and doughy compared to the Mexican tortillas that are thin and crispy. Freshly ground corn is used to make these tortillas and the women add their own flavors to the flour as well as other ingredients (bell peppers, onions, carrots, garlic). Electric blenders are not available in rural parts of Portugal so we pounded fresh corn kernels with mortar and pestle as best we could to make this soup. The Madeira recipe is a bit thicker than my recipe but just as good.*

Madera Corn Chowder Soup

6 ears of corn, kernels removed.
4 cups vanilla soy or rice milk.
1 leek or green onion, peeled, washed, sliced.
2-3 cloves garlic, minced.
1-2 tbsp. white miso.
Red pepper, saffron to taste.

Blend corn in blender/food processor.
Add leeks/onions, garlic.
Blend to smooth consistency.
Add milk and blend.

In a stainless steel pot:

Simmer on low for 30 minutes.
Remove cup of soup.

Set aside.

Dissolve miso in ½ cup of soup.
Add to the mixture.
Simmer another 15 minutes on low.
Add more milk liquids if chowder becomes too thick.
Season with pepper, saffron.
Serve.

*Corn has had many uses. Aztec Indians valued corn as much as the Spanish Conquistador Cortez's lust for gold. Many of the Aztec rituals had traditionally been dedicated to their gods. Aztec rituals were often centered on the planting and harvesting of corn or "**maize**", as the Indians refers to corn. These ceremonies were diverse and often coveted human sacrifices to insure a plentiful harvest. Today in modern times, corn throughout the Central Americas is still the primary grain. Northern American Indians incorporated corn as a medicine. Corn silk was made into a tea for urinary bladder problems or for a difficult labor. Topically, the silk relieved skin lesions and was also used as well as a symbol of wealth. With the colonization of the Americas, European settlers adapted the fermentation method of corn from the American Indians and developed "**corn whiskey**," "**corn mash**" and "**Tom's Turkey Whiskey**" which is still very popular in parts of the Appalachians Mountains today. Corn often times in its whole form as a vegetable can be difficult to digest. To resolve this dilemma, corn when used as a grain can be finely ground into a meal for easier assimilation.*

My French Onion Soup

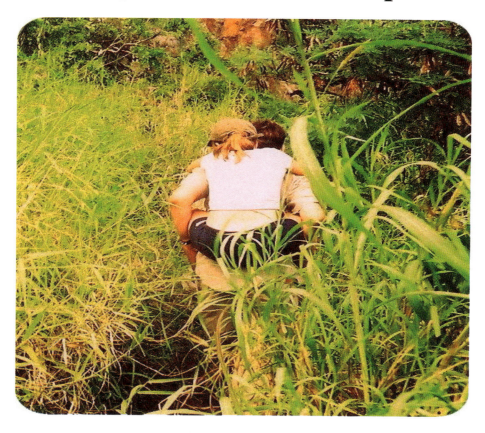

My version of a traditional **French Onion Soup** *may take a little effort to make, but the effort is well spent. The breath of caramelized onions cooking on a cold winter day whiffing throughout the house is something no one should ever miss. My son's all-time favorite, my soup takes the edge off two Hawaiian kids in the dead of winter who were used to slippers on their feet and sand between their toes. Each time I prepare this soup, I can hear my children laughing and playing as I wander in the kitchen.* **My French Onion Soup** *reminds me of what is important in life. A warm place in my heart and my children.*

My French Onion Soup

4 onions, washed, peeled, quartered.
2-3 tbsp. olive oil.
Sweet basil to taste.
Red pepper.
3 cups almond or soy vanilla milk.

Preheat oven to broil.

Place onions in a blender.
Blend for a creamier, traditional look
.

In stainless steel skillet:

Add olive oil and onions.
Slowly pile onion on top of onion.
Simmer on low 45-60 minutes.
Stir often with a wooden spoon until onions are a caramel brown.
Add milk, spices, and herbs.
Simmer on low for 30 minutes.

In oven safe soup bowls:

Place non wheat yeast bread, toasted mochi on the bottom of each soup
bowl.
Pour onion soup on top.
Crumbled sheep/goat feta on top.
Broil until a golden brown.
Serve.

*Onions are strongly antimicrobial. Believed to have originated in Egypt and migrated to East Asia onions have a long history in folk medicine as well as in culinary kitchens all throughout the world. Made into a tea for asthma or colds. Eaten raw for parasites, used in cooking to lower cholesterol are only a few of the traditional uses. Texas claims to have the sweetest onions grown anywhere, however, Maui onion farmers have claims of their own. Early Greeks rubbed onions all over their body prior to battle while ancient Egyptians valued the onion as a symbol for eternity. In traditional oriental medicine onions are included in food remedies for symptomatic coughs, colds and sore throats. In Egyptian (**Egyptian Book of the Dead**) records the onion as the symbol for the birth-death cycle of human development. Egyptians pharaohs were buried with wreaths of onions so as to revive them if not in this life then in the next. The many varieties of onions offer a wide range in tastes, flavors, textures and use in culinary kitchens and it is at the discretion of the chef on which onion is preferred in their own interpretation of my recipe.*

MY OWN ASPARAGUS SOUP

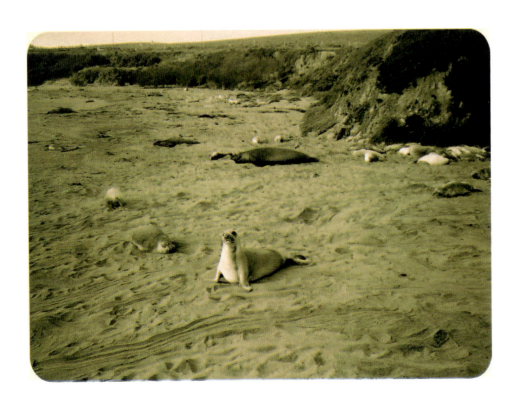

A staple table vegetable from Spain, purple, orange, yellow and red asparagus are readily available in grocery markets today. The only annoyance that my patients have expressed after preparing this asparagus dish is its very strong odor while cooking. Jerimah, a friend and patient, lives in the central coast of California and loves his asparagus steamed. In working with bouts of fatigue, I suggested that he could increase his adrenals by eating asparagus The adrenals are the foundation of health for traditional medicine. Jerimah seems to have that he took my advice.

MY OWN ASPARAGUS SOUP

1 lb. asparagus, washed, ends removed.
1 leek or green onions, sliced.
1 lb. silken tofu, cut into quarters.
Rice milk.
Black pepper.
1 bulb garlic, minced.
1 tsp. white miso.
1 tsp. each tarragon, chervil, parsley.
Olive oil/olive oil spray.
1 tsp. grated zest of lemon/lime (lemon/ lime rind).

In a steamer basket in a stainless steel pot:

Steam asparagus until soft.
Remove asparagus from heat and pot.

In a stainless steel skillet:

Sauté leeks, onions, garlic in oil until the garlic becomes a light brown.
Blend asparagus, garlic, leek/onions in a blender/ food processor until smooth.
Add tofu to the mixture.
Blend until smooth.
Add milk until desired thickness.

In a stainless steel pot:

Add spices, herbs, and miso.
Simmer in pot for 30 minutes on low.
Add olive oil and zest of lemon/lime.
Sprinkle cheese, black sesame seeds and **serve**

*This asparagus soup becomes easier to assimilate and digest by further blending and pureeing all of the ingredients. For those who find that **tofu is too heavy** for digestion or has an adverse reaction to soy products, substitution with a vegetable or grain milk is applicable. The asparagus has many traditional medicinal uses. Folk remedies have used asparagus as a diuretic, antispasmodic, anti-inflammatory, laxative and digestive stimulant. Other traditional folk medicinal uses have also included treatment for gout, arthritis and urinary tract problems. Traditional oriental herbalists use the dried roots of the asparagus for a chronic cough, to astringe the kidneys, as a tonic and to ease insomnia as well as to calm anxiety in menopausal women. Asparagus is high in magnesium. When combined with a calcium based food source such as a soy or a goat/sheep product, asparagus becomes helpful as a relaxant and nervine for fatigued muscles as well as for fatigued emotions. The fresh spears of the asparagus while cooking produce a strong odor and color the urine after ingesting due to its very high concentration of chlorophyll.*

My Own Papaya Curried Soup

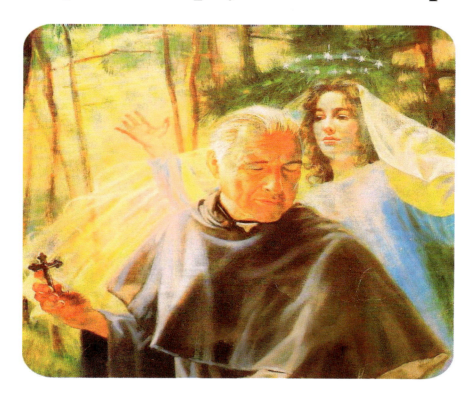

Fr. Peter Mary Rookey of St. Michael's International Compassionate Ministry is my inspiration. Father has always taken the time to listen and bless me on many of my most difficult challenges. At the age of 96, Father is still active holding daily services as well as giving counsel at St. Michael's. Driving to Austin, Texas I talking my way through the desert with Father when a highway patrol officer passed me and waved. As is the custom in Hawaii, I waved back and as I did so I noticed my odometer's reading. God Bless you Father for always keeping me safe in foreign lands.

My Own Papaya Curried Soup

2-3 green ripe papayas cut in half seeds removed.
4 cups almond milk.
2-3 limes.
Masala red curry.
Mint leaves.
Cinnamon.

Scoop papaya meat into a blender/ food processor.
Blend until smooth.

In a stainless steel pot.

Place papaya meat in pot.
Add milk.
Heat on low.
Add limes juice.
Stir gently.
Remove a small amount of liquid from pot.
Combine with curry.
Dissolve curry in liquid.
Pour in serving bowl.
Place mint/sprinkle cinnamon on top.
Serve.

*Papayas are tropical fruit that require a warm climate in which to grow. Papayas are cultivated in Asia, Africa, Mexico and Hawaii. The papaya has many commercial, culinary and medicinal uses. Examples of commercial uses are as a protein enzyme for contact lenses and digestive enzymes for stomach disorders. On Maui, sugar mill workers introduced me to their use of the papaya. A tablespoon of the papaya seeds were chewed for indigestion or intestinal worms. Boiling the rind of a green papaya in water and drink it as a tea to treat a stomach ache. The peel and the meat of the papaya are left over night to remove freckles on the face. Throughout the world there is now papaya salsa, papaya cream, papaya smoothies, papaya whole, sliced or stewed. The papaya is a very unique fruit in that the peel of the papaya is acidic in nature, the meat is neutral and the seeds are alkalizing. My auntie prefers the large Mexican papaya to the small Hawaiian papaya. I can still hear her saying when I gave her a Solo local papaya , **"at home we feed this to the pigs"**.*

Lemongrass Rice Noodle Soup

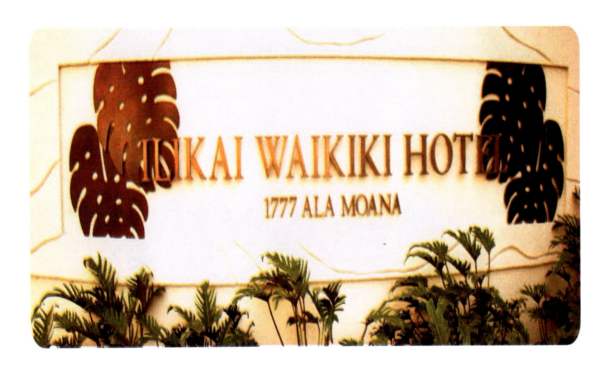

Lemongrass is a very beautiful flowering herb used in decorations as well culinary practices throughout Asia particularly Thailand. The manager of the Ilikai Hotel in Honolulu, Hawaii during the late nineteen sixties enjoyed this recipe. Now living on the coast of New Jersey, David shared his memories as I cooked in his kitchen. The aromas of a time long gone wafted through David's kitchen as we worked through his program treating an elevated PSA. Ten days later with a clean bill of health and a lab report to prove it, David went fishing out on his river in June of 2010 and I do believe he may be there still be there.

Lemongrass Rice Noodle Soup

6 carrots, sliced.
1 turnip, washed, peeled, quartered.
1-2 leeks or green onions, peeled, washed, sliced into moons.
1-2 zucchini, quarter.
1 cup fresh peas, shelled.
1 rind of lemon/lime grated.
1-2 tbsp. lemongrass or juice of one lemon/lime.
1-2 garlic cloves, minced.
Fresh ginger, grated.
Red crushed pepper to taste.
Olive oil.
1 package rice vermilion bean noodle, thread style.

In a stainless steel skillet:

Sauté carrots, turnip, leek/onions, zucchini, peas in olive oil.

In a stainless steel pot:

Combine sauté vegetables with 4-6 cups of water.
Add herbs.
Simmer for 30-40 minutes.
Add lemon/lime rind.
Add noodles to soup.
Simmer for additional 10 min.
Serve.

*A fast growing tall perennial grass, lemongrass was originally cultivated in India, Thailand and Sri Lanka. Used extensively in Thai soups and curries lemongrass gives a light aromatic flavor to everything it is cooked with. Lemongrass is found more and more frequently in supermarkets in North America and Europe. An important medicinal and culinary herb in South and Central America, Asia and the Caribbean, lemongrass is known as "**fever grass**" for its healing properties in treating cholera and its associated fevers. India's Ayurveda practioners will use lemongrass in the form of a tea for colds, flues and other respitory conditions. Lemongrass also treats pain arising from indigestion, rheumatism, and nerve conditions. Researchers have found the refreshing fragrance from the lemongrass to reduce headaches, irritability and to prevent drowsiness. Lemongrass is nontoxic but can cause sensitivity with some individuals. Traditionally, throughout Asia, an infusion of tea is made from the stalks of the lemongrass and 1-4 cups were drunk daily for coughs, colds, indigestion, menstrual disorders and headaches.*

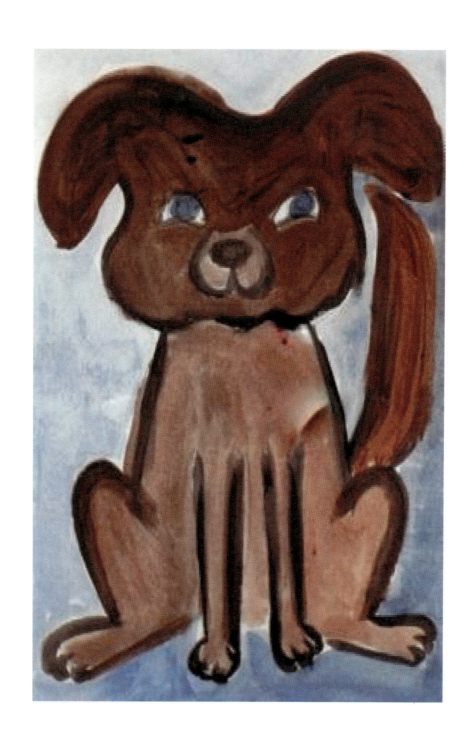

MAIN COURSE

Alicia's Macadamia Nut Pesto

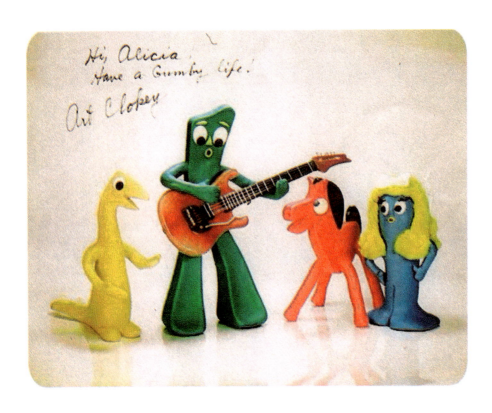

On my eighteenth birthday my mom gave me my first mini food processor and this recipe. It was my first year in college, on my own and away from friends, family and Hawaii. I was living in the dorms at the University of San Francisco suffering through the bland cafeteria foods. With my mom's easy recipe of **Macadamia Nut Pesto** *I was able to make it through the first year. I put the pesto on everything and even ate it as is. I eventually started cooking many of mom's recipes for myself and my roommates as well. I now teach in Japan and* **Macadamia Nut Pesto** *is still my favorite of all mom's recipes.*

Alicia's Macadamia Nut Basil Pesto

1 cup macadamia nuts.
1 cup goat/sheep Romano Pecorino, grated.
2 cups fresh sweet basil.
1 cup fresh parsley, heads.
2-6 garlic cloves mince
1 ½ cups olive oil.

Chop nuts in blender/ food processor.
Blend until smooth.
Gradually add basil, parsley, garlic, olive oil.
Blend until smooth.
Add cheese.
Blend until desired consistency.

For a thicker pesto add more cheese, for thinner add more oil.

Macadamia nuts originate in Australia and are commercially cultivated in Hawaii, Mexico, South Africa, China and other parts of the world. Commercial use as well as the health benefits of the macadamia nut are constantly in scientific review. Macadamia nuts can be ground into a flour and used in gluten wheat free recipes, into a butter and cold pressed into an oil where it is used to moisturize skin as well as for cooking oil. The Big Island of Hawaii has the largest Mac farms in Hawaii and produces some of highest quality of macadamias in the world.. There are a variety of uses for the macadamia nut ranging from cosmetics to coffee, cooking, liquors, as well as in farming. With a high protein concentration per nut (around 9% per nut), macadamias provide an excellent choice for athletes as well as college students on the run. Helpful in diets that incorporate low cholesterol foods, macadamia nuts provide a healthy choice.

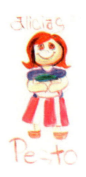

American Macro Artichoke Enchiladas

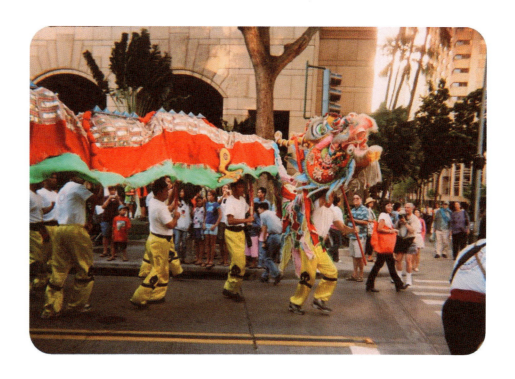

*I was introduced to enchiladas while working in Los Angeles Chinatown in California. The true Mexican enchiladas proved to be too spicy for me and the cheeses made my nose stuffy. But I liked them. Traditional enchiladas are made with a corn wrapper. I replaced the corn wrapper with a spelt or rice tortilla and introduced this version to my family and patients. Until the 1980's, tofu was confined to Asian communities and health food stores. Eventually, dairy free products as well as tofu became available in many mainstream markets. For this recipe I added the artichoke heart and it became the signature vegetable for my **American Macro Enchiladas.***

American Macro Artichoke Enchiladas

12 corn, spelt or rice tortillas.
3-6 tbsp. olive oil.
1/3 cup spelt flour.
1 ½ cups vegetable broth.
½ cup nondairy sour cream.
1 green chili diced, deseeded.
2 ½ cup tofu, cubed.
1 leek or green onion, diced.
1 lb. artichoke hearts, chopped.
Sheep/goat Monterey cheese, graded.

Preheat oven to 350 degrees

In a stainless steel skillet:

Heat oil on low
Add tortillas to skillet.
Heat each tortilla briefly on both sides.
Remove tortillas from heat.
Set aside on a plate.

Sauce:

In a stainless steel skillet:

Heat oil on low.
Add flour to pan.

Blend.

Add broth.
Cook on very low until thickened.
Stir often.
Add sour cream, chilies.
Cook on low.
Stir.
Add tofu, onion, artichoke into sauce.

In an oven safe casserole dish:

Place tortillas side by side.
Place all ingredients in each tortillas.
Roll up tortillas.
Sprinkle cheese over tortilla and mixture.
Top with remaining sauce and cheese.
Bake for 25 minutes, or until heated through.
Serve.

*Corn originated in Central America. It is the primary grain that was utilized by the many indigenous culture. Made into many products, corn can be ground into a flour, eaten raw, cold pressed into an oil, cooked in soups, stews or as a compliment to other meals. Aztec Indians traditionally made a flat unleavened bread from ground corn, water and lime which have become the tortillas of today. Tortillas are known as the "**bread of Mexico**" and are used as a substitute for the fork, spoon, plate and bowl. The famous Spanish conquistador Cortez discovered more than gold when he arrived in the Central Americas. The conquistadores discovered a unique civilization years ahead of their own culture that was based on corn. Ceremonies devoted to their **Corn God**, marriages, births and deaths were deeply rooted around the cultivation and harvesting of corn. To this day, Central Americans still eat many of the traditional foods from the Aztec Indians that is based on corn. Commercially, corn is being researched as a safe alternative to petroleum products, packaging material as well as building resources.*

American Macro Cornbread

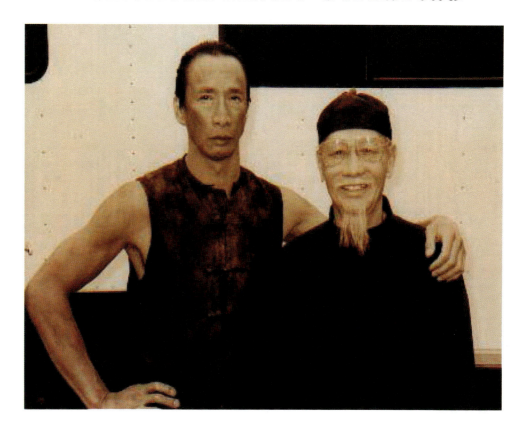

One of my oldest friend in Hawaii is Roland Nip. Originally my family attorney, Roland over the last 20 years has moved onto becoming a very visible actor and accomplished tai qi instructor. I first met Roland when he closed his law practice to assist with hospice care for his mother. Over the year, Roland's health had declined while working as a public defender resulting in mitral valve prolapse. Today, Roland is in complete recovery. "All attorneys are actors", Roland quotes. I am not sure exactly what that means, but Roland is finally playing the part he was born to play. **Himself.**

American Macro Cornbread

1 ½ cup spelt flour.
1 cup cornmeal.
1 cup fresh corn kernels.
1 leek or red onion, peeled, washed, sliced.
2-4 tsp. baking powder.
½ cup olive oil.
1 ½ cup rice or soy milk.
Nondairy yogurt.
1 cup agave, honey, or sucanat.

Preheat oven to 350 degrees.

Lightly oil and flour an oven safe baking dish.
Sift dry ingredients in one bowl.
Mix in milk, yogurt and oil.
Blend.
Add more milk if needed until batter is smooth.
Fold in corn kernels.

For a sweeter corn bread:

Add 1 cup agave, honey or sucanat.
Bake at 350 degrees for 30-35 minutes until a knife cleanly sears the corn bread when placed through the center.
Serve.

*Corn meal is the coarsely ground grain from corn. Corn meal became popular in the Americas during the depression in the 1920's when flour and it products became scarce. One of the problems resulting from over consumption of corn products was a condition called "**pellagra**" a skin disease that resulted from a deficiency particularly in B vitamins (**Merck Manual 2004**).The addition of lime and water when using corn meal as demonstrated by South American Indians proved that it was not the corn that caused pellagra, but the manner in which it was prepared. Corn has a place in Native American history throughout all the Americas. Ceremonies of birth, weddings and death are well documented as well as the medicinal usages for corn. Corn meal has been touted in folk remedies for fungal infections when made into a paste and applied on the infection site, for hypertension with its nutritional support of the amino acid lysine along with B vitamins which help maintain the integrity of the heart muscle. One of the largest cultivated crops in the world, corn is also being viewed as an industrial alternative to petroleum based energy products such as oil, petrol, food packaging, hair coloring, and more.*

Artichokes with Goat Ricotta and Basil

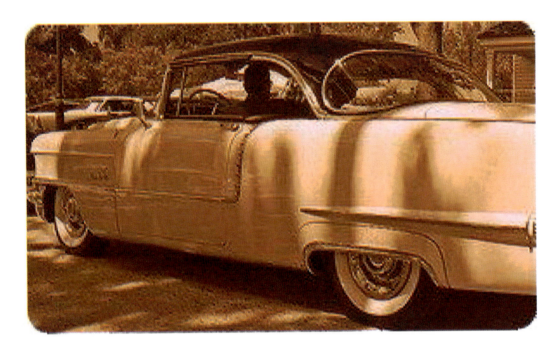

*I had always avoided the artichoke. Classified as a thistle, even animals avoided the plant. Not much to look at, difficult to prepare as well as difficult to eat, I thought of the artichoke as **"God's Joke of Nature"**. My minimal experience with the artichoke was sitting at a kitchen table while the leafs of the artichoke were dipped in melted butter or in mayonnaise. Not very appealing. An opportunity presented itself when an Italian woman shared recipes with me from of her family. This recipe is a complement to Alma, her recipe and her pink Cadillac. I will always remember Alma as one of the great women of the Central Coast of California and dedicate this recipe to her.*

Artichokes with Goat Ricotta and Basil

4 lg. artichokes.
2 tbsp. lemon juice.
1 cup goat ricotta cheese.
1 cup goat/sheep Romano pecorino.
1 cup basil, chopped.
½ teaspoon ground pepper.
Olive Oil.
1 garlic bulb, minced.
Macadamia nuts, chopped.

Preheat oven to 375 degrees.

Rinse artichokes, cut stems and top third of petals.
Cut artichokes in half lengthwise.
Arrange in 2 baking dishes, cut side facing down.
Add water to fill halfway.
Squeeze lemon juice over artichokes.
Cover baking dish.
Place in oven.
Bake 30 minutes until leaves easily are removed.

In a bowl:

Combine cheeses, olive oil, basil, garlic, ground pepper.
Set aside.
When artichokes are done.
Remove from oven.

Drain excess liquid from baking dishes.

Turn over artichoke.

Remove fuzzy artichoke center, and inner leaves.

Drizzle artichoke with olive oil.

Sprinkle artichokes with macadamia nuts, pecorino.

Spoon ricotta mixture into each artichoke halves.

Return to oven.

Bake until cheese is lightly brown.

Serve.

*Artichokes migrated from Northern Africa to Europe where it was first grown as a perennial plant in England (**Wikipedia**). The leaves and core or "heart" of the artichoke can be boiled, steamed or deep fried. It is advisable when cooking the artichoke not to cover them. The artichoke is highly acidic and releases a volatile gas when heated which can be toxic. By not covering the pot or pan this gas will disperse into the air unharmed. Traditional oriental practitioners incorporated the artichoke as a digestive aide for stomach aches and in its assistance for the body's production of bile. Health stores retail prepared artichoke capsules for the use in reduction of cholesterol. A very useful thistle, the artichoke leaves, its heart and even the stems are edible. Roadside gardeners often will plant the artichoke for their beautiful purple flowers and easy maintained. The water that remains from boiling an artichoke can be applied as a broth for cooking grains such as rice or millet. Artichokes are traditionally marinated in olive oil in Greek and Italian cultures.*

Feta Stuffed Sweet Bell Peppers

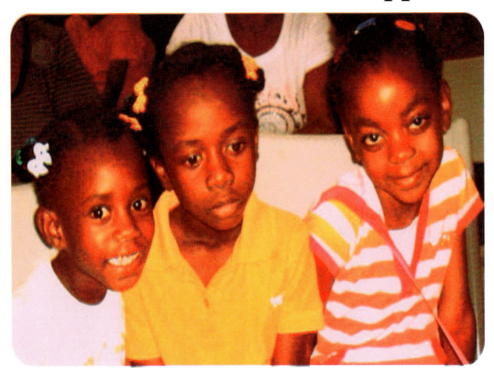

I prefer sweet red bell peppers to all other peppers. This recipe was the favorite of one of my Hepatitis C patients. It is often difficult to diagnose hepatitis. Coronary heart disease, diabetes, bile duct conditions, and hypertension often complicate a diagnosis for Hepatitis. With a correct diagnosis effective treatments can proceed. While working in the Caribbean, I visited an orphanage in Antigua where many of the children were suffering with this terrible disease. I told them a story about a baby bell pepper and her journey through the garden to become a swan and who flew away to live happier ever after.
This recipe is for the children.

Feta Stuffed Sweet Bell Peppers

2 sweet red, yellow or green bell peppers, washed, de-seeded.
2-3 cups cooked millet, or brown rice.
4-6 carrots, sliced.
1 leek or green onion, sliced.
1 garlic bulb, minced.
1 cup fresh peas.
2-3tbsp. olive oil.
Goat/sheep feta, crumbled.
Sheep/goat Pecorino Romano cheese, grated.

Preheat oven at 350 degrees.

In a stainless steel pot place a steamer basket:

Fill with water to bottom of steamer basket.
Fill peppers with water.
Place in peppers, carrots and peas.
Steam peppers, carrots, peas in water until soft, yet firm.
Drain water from pot.
Remove peppers from pot.
Place peppers in a casserole dish.

In stainless steel skillet.

Sauté leeks, onions, garlic in olive oil until onions are a clear opaque color.
Remove from heat

Set aside

In a bowl:

Mix grains, vegetables together.
Stuff grains, vegetables into peppers.

Place in an oven safe casserole dish.

Top with cheeses.
Bake at 350 degrees for 15 minutes.
Broil until a golden brown.
Garnish with parsley and lemon slices.
Serve.

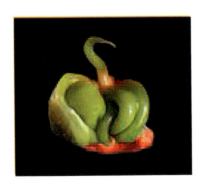

The Bell Pepper is a member of the pepper family and is rich in Vitamin C and Vitamin A. The red bell peppers are really green peppers that have become more mature through aging. These sweet peppers are not hot as their cousins the "red peppers" which produce Caspian, a heating element found in cayenne and saffron. The origin of the bell pepper is not adequately known though today "bells" are cultivated all over the world. The use of millet in this recipe provides additional vitamins and a form of protein that is easily digested. My teacher Dr. Hok Chi Tse, a gynecologist from Macau told me that in China women were given fifty pounds of millet after they had given birth to regain their strength and health. Millet is a small round yellow to brown grain that requires a dry climate for cultivation until harvest. Olive oil consists of essential fatty acids called Omega 3, 6 and 9. These omegas help to maintain the integrity of the body's muscles and retain the smooth texture of the skin. Olive oil in combination with protein from the cheeses, B vitamins from millet and the vitamins and minerals from the bell peppers, make this recipe a complete meal.

Gingered Tofu Vegetables and Miriam

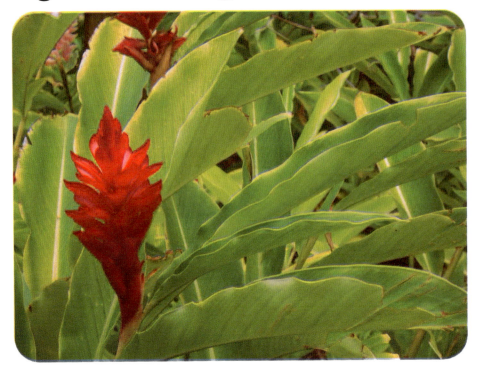

*Ginger is more valuable in the Orient than its weight in gold. Beautiful in appearance, ginger can grow to a height of 6 feet and more. My student and friend, **Miriam** tells me that this is her favorite of all my recipe. Marian was traveling in New Zealand when she experienced heart palpitations and immediately flew to Hawaii to see me. Once in Hawaii, Miriam became my "**taste pilot**" as well as my patient. A brilliant acupuncturist in Santa Barbara, California as well as a mother, wife and an established artist, Marian includes my recipes in many of the meals she prepares for her family and friends.*

Gingered Tofu with Vegetables and Miriam

1 extra firm tofu sliced, cubed.
1 leek or green onion, peeled, washed, sliced.
3-6 inch ginger root, grated.
2-3 tbsp. Braggs Amino Acids.
1-3 tbsp. olive oil.
½ cup water.
Carrots, zucchini, cauliflower peas, bean pods, etc.

Preheat oven to 350 degrees.

In a bowl:

Marinate all vegetables in Braggs, olive oil over night.

In an oven safe casserole dish:

Add vegetables with marinate.
Bake for 45 minutes.
Add water as needed so mixture will not dry out.
Serve over rice or noodles.

Radix zingerberis, ginger, is a perennial plant that prefers cultivation in warmer climates. The roots from the ginger plant are used in cooking or herbal preparations. Buried deep within the ground the ginger roots can grow in length of 3 feet and longer. Ginger shoots are the young immature sprouts of the plant used in decorations as well as a food source. Fresh ginger can be a light pink in color to a red hue. Delicate in flavor, I prefer using fresh Hawaiian ginger with stir fries and aged Asian ginger for stronger dishes such as curries and soups. Ginger has traditional use in oriental medicine as a digestive aide as well as a calmative. Warming and slightly spicy, oriental herbalists include ginger to disperse **"phlegm"** and **"mucous"** from the lungs giving breath and adding length and depth. Prepared as a tea, ginger has been used to warm a cold, ease a cough, relax the chest and stop a stomach ache. Ginger can be made into a candy, added to soups, used in cooking oils or added with a carrier oil to draw out tired muscles in Japanese Kanpo formula. Very popular in folk remedies throughout the world, ginger's is still used as a spice as well as a medicinal herb

.

Golden Beets with Marinated Carrots

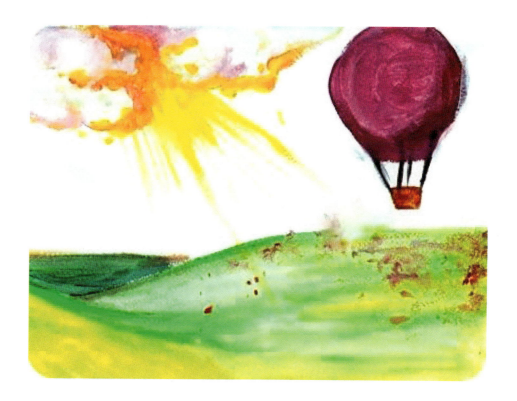

A golden beet surrounded with sparkling carrots, drenched and bathed in extra virgin olive oil and garlic with a sprinkle of black sesame seeds is the alluring dish a Maryland patient inspired. After staining myself and the countertop of the kitchen I was working on with red beet juice I decided to find an alternative with the same nutritional value as the red beet, but with less mess. I wandered through a farmers' marker in despair until I glimpsed a beautiful smooth hairless beet so named the **"Golden Beet."** *My patient was ecstatic, her fibroids in remission and her countertops.*

Golden Beets with Marinated Carrots

1 lb. golden beets, quartered, beet tops removed, washed.
4-6 carrots, sliced.
6 baby Boc Choy leaves.
1 leek or green onion, peeled, washed, sliced.
1 garlic bulb, minced.
1 cup raw macadamia nuts.
Rosemary sprigs garlic powder.
Extra virgin olive oil.
Sheep/goat feta, crumbled.

Preheat oven to 350 degrees.

Put on latex free kitchen gloves.

In a stainless steel pot place a steamer basket:

Place beets, carrots in basket.
Steam on high.
Remove from heat when beets are soft.
Cool beets and carrots.
Rub off the beet skin with vegetable brush.

In a stainless steel skillet:

Toss boc choy, leeks, garlic in olive oil

In an oven safe casserole dish:

Place boc choy on the bottom.
Layer beets, carrots, leeks and garlic on top.
Mix olive oil with garlic powder and rosemary.
Drizzle olive oil mixture over vegetables

Sprinkle macadamia nuts on top of the vegetables.
Bake for 30 minutes.
Remove from oven.
Add cheeses.
Broil until golden brown.
Serve.

*Whenever cooking beets it is best if the tops of the beets are removed leaving 1 inch above the tuber. With boiling or steaming, place the whole beet in the pot and when finished, rub or peel the skin off and cut away the remaining stem and root. With roasting, first peel the skin then remove the remaining stem and root. Always wear gloves when working with beets. Be sure to wear an apron as well and cover the area you will be preparing the beets on so as not to change the color of the counter or yourself. Beets are considered an estrogen vegetable by practitioners of oriental medicine included in diets for hormone related conditions in pre and post women. In many traditional folk remedies, the beet is the signature vegetable for women. Some believe that the beet is shaped in the form of a women's uterus and is helpful for bleeding disorders during menopause as the beet will also "bleed" when it matures. Homeopathic philosophy where "**Like treats Like**" can be applied to the role of the beet by the of revitalization women hormonal system as a phytoestrogen.*

Grandma Evey's Long Beans and Rice

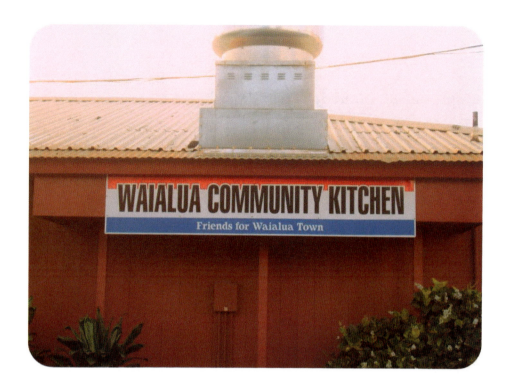

*Long beans are native to the Philippines, Thailand and other parts of Asia. All my P.I. aunties have their own way of preparing long beans. My favorite is **Grandma Evey's Long Bean** recipe. Before World War11, Evelyn was a Kahuku plantation nurse. Her husband Frank, was a train engineer for the sugar companies on Oahu. Our constant conversation over 20 years of friendship was who wrote the music, "**I heard it through the grapevine**", which I can never remember. I do remember that her favorite group was the **Ink Spots.** When I prepare this recipe I can hear their songs as well as Grandma Evey's stories.*

Grandma Evey's Long Beans and Rice

1 lb. green beans.
1 leek or green onion, peeled, washed, sliced.
2-6 garlic cloves, minced.
Sliced almonds.
2-4 tbsp. olive oil.

In a stainless steel skillet:

Sauté onions/garlic in oil.
Add green beans and almonds.
Simmer until crisp and tender.
Serve with rice.

Green Beans are immature young legumes still in their pod. High in magnesium and chlorophyll, green beans are included in diets for hypertension, elevated cholesterol and diabetes. Hawaii has a high population of diabetic's acquired, adult onset and juvenile. There is a wonderful individual here in the Islands that have devoted his time to educating as well as working with islanders who suffer from diet related conditions on the coast of Waianae, Oahu. The use of long green beans as well as other local vegetables familiar to Hawaii is incorporated with meal planning for these individuals as well as others. To address the health concerns of our state, many restaurants offer meals prepared especially for diet related conditions. Long green beans are often within many of these meals. As an effort to control Hawaii's increasing population of obesity, a task force was developed by Hawaiian legislators aimed at creating better food choices within our schools as well as our medical facilities. Many of Hawaii's local restaurants have created "healthy menus" for their patrons which include salt free, diabetic desserts, low cholesterol and gluten free meals.

Hand Held Nori Roll

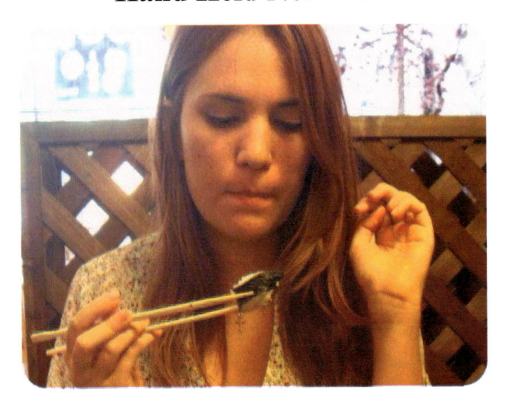

*Introducing patients to macrobiotic foods and its lifestyle proved to be something of a challenge. Many individuals first experience to Asian foods is through the Japanese "sushi" which is a sheet of seaweed (**nori**) wrapped around white rice. My patients were comfortable with the traditional sushi so for them I developed my **Hand Held Nori Rolls**. My nori rolls have a macro flair of grains, avocado, salsa, jalapeño peppers, ginger, beans and anything else that can fit into my roll. These nori rolls are larger than traditional sushi rolls making chop sticks easier to use or you can just hold them in your hands.*

Hand Held Nori Rolls

Nori Seaweed Sheets.
1 cup cooked brown rice, millet or any other desired grain.
Raw carrots, daikon radish, cucumber, zucchini, shredded.
1 avocado.
Red leaf lettuce.
Steamed veggies, if desired.
Tofu, cubed.
Braggs, olive oil, garlic powder lemon/lime, salsa if desired.

On a clean cutting board:

Place desired vegetables, rice on the nori sheet.
Drizzle desired flavor onto vegetables (olive oil, Braggs, etc.)
Roll nori sheet with vegetables, grain inside end to end.
Moisten edges with water to maintain a firm roll.
Serve.

Nori is the most familiar sea vegetable within the United States made popular by the many "sushi restaurants". High in protein, nori is a pressed sheet of seaweed that ranges from light green to a dark black and used in soups, salads, or rolled up to hold rice and vegetables. In Hawaii, nori rolls are called **Plum rolls***. In Scotland a similar form of the Japanese nori is* **"laver"** *deep Atlantic sea kelp. Today the most abundant supply of fresh edible sea vegetable products is harvested off the Eastern Coast of Maine and Norway. Our oceans are becoming compromised with higher incidences of pollution. The result is a steady decline of all sea vegetation. As seaweeds have a variety of medicinal usages, their decline will hamper research in many areas particularly endocrinology and cardiology. Traditionally, Asian medicine included sea vegetables in food formula to aide metabolism, dissolve nodules, support the immune system, increase vision, reduce blood pressure and more.*

Hallelujah Cashew Asparagus

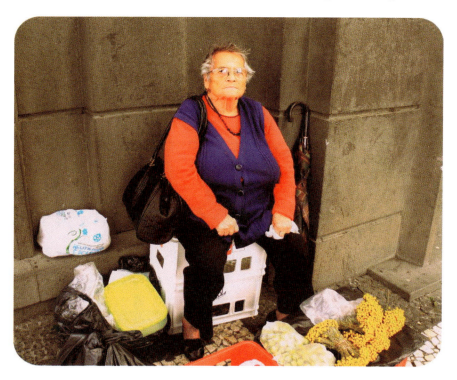

On December 15, 2008 Hawaii's Honolulu Advertiser began addressing domestic violence aggressively for the first time in the state's history. The Advertiser began publishing daily for 6 weeks stories of domestic violence within all Hawaiian Islands. Hawaii's domestic violence ranks as number 1 in the United States today. With public awareness and active participation within our legislation there is hope. **Hallelujah Cashew** *was developed from my own personal experience in the fight against domestic violence. The Advertiser's news releases are a small part of a larger movement within Hawaii to bring change and the necessary attention to stop domestic violence.*

Hallelujah Cashew Asparagus

1lb. fresh asparagus, washed.
1 cup roasted cashews.
Olive oil.
½ tsp. red pepper flakes.
Cayenne pepper to taste.
Béarnaise sauce (recipe below).

Trim 2 inches off the ends of asparagus.
Place asparagus.

In steamer basket in stainless steel pot with water.

Steam asparagus until tender.
Remove from heat.
Drain water from pot.
Set aside.
Toast cashews in olive oil in stainless steel skillet.
Add spices.
Arrange asparagus on a serving platter.
Pour Béarnaise sauce over asparagus.
Sprinkle with crushed cashews.
Serve.

Béarnaise Sauce

White and black pepper.
2-3 tbsp. lemon juice.
6 cloves garlic, minced.
Silken tofu, cubed.
Blend ingredients together in a blender /food processor until smooth.

In stainless steel pot:

Heat on low.
Stir.
Serve.

Asparagus is a very beautiful and fragile plant. Traditional oriental practitioners have used dried and prepared asparagus root as a tonic for the lungs and the kidneys. Originally cultivated in parts of Europe, asparagus plants do very well in subtropical or tropical climates. It takes 2-3 years for an asparagus's root system to mature. The male plants grow to heights of 15 centimeters above ground after the second year and it is at this time that harvesting will produce a sweet tender frond. Folk medicine has utilized asparagus as a laxative, sedative, antispasmodic, and a tonic for the heart.

Domestic violence is the true #1 disease process in the United States today. Generations of domestic violence cases crowd every state's court rooms, hospitals, schools, and work places. There is no discrimination in color or economics with domestic violence. A disease that covers a broad spectrum left untreated becomes contagious spreading from one family member to the next.

Hawaii is one of the last states in the nation *to pass laws to effectively prosecute offenders of Domestic Violence and protect their victims.*

I want to give a **thank you** *to all the social workers, school psychologist, CSEA, and CPS employees.*

George Moore at CPS on the Big Island.

A loving thanks to all law enforcement agents for all their efforts in **assisting to take back the night.**

In March of 2009, Hawaii was reported as #1 for Domestic Violence in the United States.

By the end of 2011, Hawaii is still #1 for domestic Violence nationwide.

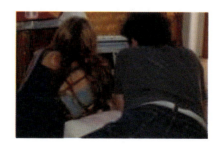

Italian French Bean Sauté

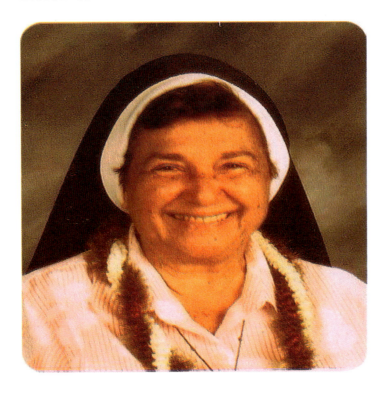

One of my favorite people is Sister Margaret Antoine. Born and raised on the Big Island of Hawaii, Sister Margaret was the Vice Principal of Saint Francis School for Girls of when my daughter attended. I dearly love Sister Margaret and it should be noted that Sister Margret gave great input with the editing of the first edition of **Inspiration for Health**. *Sister Margaret is a very independent individual so much so that in JFK's airport in New York at the baggage claims she refused to let anyone assist her in retrieving her luggage. As a result she had a free ride on the conveyor belt.*

Italian French Bean Sauté

4 tbsp. extra virgin olive oil.
2 -6 garlic cloves, minced.
1 lb. French green beans, trimmed, cut.
2 leeks or green onions, peeled, washed, sliced.
6 tbsp. water or vegetable broth.
1 cup baby carrots, whole.
1 tsp. dried basil.
1 tsp. thyme.
6 fresh basil leaves, shredded.
1 cup sheep/goat Romano Pecorino cheese, grated.
Bragg's amino acids or wheat free tamari to taste.

Preheat oven to 350 degrees.

In a stainless steel skillet:

Heat olive oil.
Add garlic and leeks.
Simmer on low until tender.
Add green beans.
Stir garlic, leeks and green beans.
Add vegetable broth/water.
Simmer on low.
Stir in baby carrots, dry basil and thyme.
Simmer on low.
Stir in fresh basil leaves.
Remove from heat.
Place in an oven safe casserole dish.
Sprinkle cheese over vegetables.Heat for 15- 25 minutes until green beans are crisp at the ends.

*Greens beans belong to the Fabaceae family of legumes. The "green bean" refers to the beans within the pods which are young and unripe. The green bean is a vine that will grows with the assistance of a trestle or some other means of sturdy support. The vines are strong and if left unattended can over years, uproot and destroy standing structures such as stone walls, fences, etc. The vines can creep up any stationary structure such as a tree devouring the trunk. Composed mainly of cellulose, water and magnesium green beans are useful as a natural form of fiber and also as a diuretic. With its high concentration of magnesium it will combine well with a calcium base food source aiding in its assimilation. Probably the most famous green bean is from **Jack and the Bean Stalk** where a young farmer trades his milk cow for a hand full of magic beans. Used in many Asian dishes as it combines well with anything, the green bean has been used for hypertension, cardiovascular disease and to lower cholesterol in food based formulas by traditional oriental practice.*

Hawaiian Macro Polenta

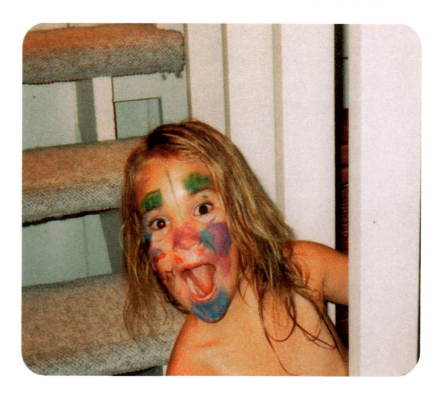

One out of three individuals in the state of Hawaii will accumulate enough sun exposure in childhood to develop topical melanoma as adults. Hawaii is best known for its recreational fun in the sun. Activities include water sports, hiking, biking, hunting and running. When my daughter was three years old she had a small blemish on her chin. She was diagnosed with a pyrogenic granuloma. Granulomas usually occur at sites of trauma and can become aggravated with sun exposure .Her granuloma was removed with minor surgery and without any anesthesia. From that day hence , my daughter resembled a kabuki dancer covered from head to toe in sunscreen.

Hawaiian Macro Polenta

1-2 cups of organic yellow corn grits (polenta).
4 cups water (add more if needed).
1 leek or green onion, peeled, washed, sliced.
1 cup fresh corn.
1 zucchini, quartered.
1-2 carrots, sliced.
2-4 tbsp. olive oil.
1 garlic bulb, minced.
1-1_ cup goat/sheep Pecorino Romano cheese, grated.
Goat/sheep feta, crumbled.

Preheat oven to 350 degrees:

In stainless steel pot:

Boil 4 cups of water.
Reduce heat.
Add polenta, vegetables, and leeks/onions to pot.
Simmer on low for 30 minutes.
Stir often. (If mixture dries, add water)
Remove from heat.

Mix oil, garlic, Romano pecorino into polenta.
Place in an oven safe casserole or pie dish.
Top with crumbled feta.
Bake at 350 degrees for 30 minutes.
Bring oven temperature to broil.
Broil until cheese is brown and toasted.
Serve.

*The Mayan Indians considered corn a gift from their Gods and believed that man was made of corn (Popol Vuh, the sacred text of the Maya). It is the essential grain in Central America (corn tortilla, tamale) and when combined with beans produce a complete protein meal. Traditional medicinal uses for corn include use as an antifungal, a diuretic, for herpes zoster and as a cold remedy. Corn silk made into a tea is given for urinary track inflammation and to ease women's labor. The husks of the corn when ground into a powder are used in animal feed products as are the cobs. Ground into flour or a meal, corn kernels can be dried for chicken feed as well as roasted and salted for human consumption. Corn can be cold pressed to produce oil that is used in cooking, and converted for commercial use as an energy alternative for fuel as well as in the manufacturing of biodegradable food packaging. Corn is **coarsely** ground for polenta**, finely** ground into flour, **blended** into a paste, or **popped** for the movies the use of corn is countless. Today, the versatility of corn is being redefined for today's environmental challenges.*

Kathleen's Spicy Black Beans with Fiery Red Peppers

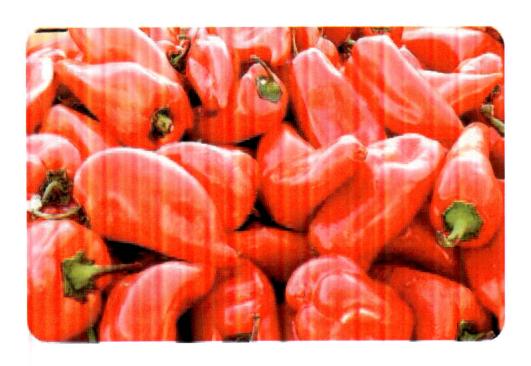

At eight years old, I was put to work in the cotton fields of North Carolina. By the end of the day the owners of the farm realized that I was not a "cotton picker" and moved me where little people like me would throw tobacco leaves onto a moving conveyer belt while adults cut and wrapped the leaves. In the fields, I was always hungry. Kathleen, a twelve year old Cherokee reservation girl, introduced me to **"beans in a pot"**. *These beans were cooked in the fields over open flames all day long for the workers. When I prepare this meal I can hear Kathleen's infectious laughter as we ran between the tobaccos stalks stealing beans.*

Kathleen's Spicy Black Beans with fiery Red Peppers

1 3 inch kelp, washed.
1 cup dry black beans, washed, rinsed.
3-4 cups water.
2 leeks or red onions, sliced.
4-7 inch ginger root, minced
1 bulb garlic, minced.
2 green/red chilies, seeds removed, sliced.
1 zucchini, quartered.
1 cup carrots, shredded.
2 red jalapeno peppers.
Braggs Amino, wheat free tamari.
1-3 tbsp. olive oil.
Parsley.

In a crock:

Place kelp at the bottom.
Add beans.
Cover beans with water.
Slow cook overnight.
Drain water.
Discard kelp.

.

Remove beans from crock pot.

In stainless steel pot.

Add beans.
Season with Braggs to taste.

115

In a stainless steel skillet:

In 1-3 TBSB of olive oil:

Sauté garlic, onions, ginger, chilies until onions are transparent.
Char peppers in a skillet whole until black.

With a fork:

Place peppers in a paper bag.
Fold the top of the back to close.
Steam peppers in the paper bag.

Allow to cool.

Unroll paper bag and remove peppers.

Wearing gloves:

Remove the skin from the peppers by peeling back the skin.
Remove the seeds with a spoon.
Combine peppers, vegetables and beans.

Garnish with parsley.
Serve.

*Black beans are warm weather crops that originated in Southern Mexico and Central America. Black beans have since migrated to all parts of the world. There has even been a black bean that has been cultivated for its spicy flavor, the **"Wasabi Black Bean"** from China. Comparative research has shown the black bean to have similar nutritional values as the soybean when used for lowering elevated cholesterol. However, the black bean's protein levels are much higher than the soybean and its fat levels are lower. Traditional Oriental practitioners believe the black bean to influence the kidney and adrenals functions and to aid women through menopause by increasing estrogen production. Black beans can be boiled, sprouted, mashed and made into flour for baking. Black beans are made into a sauce and served over mung beans with rice and given after childbirth as a tonic for the mother and as a preventative against **"bed fever"**. In Honolulu's Chinatown, black beans are made into a pastry covered in black sugar and eaten in the New Year for prosperity and good luck.*

Lotus Root Stuffed with Almond

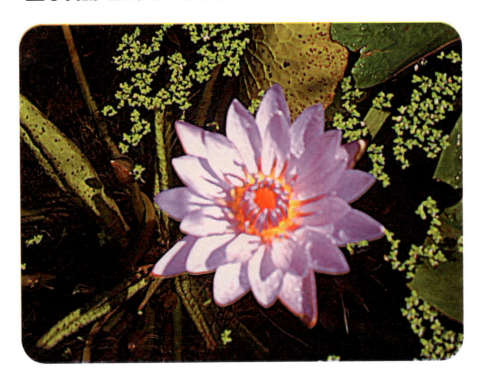

The Lotus plant has many medicinal usages. The root, dried and ground into a powder, is prepared as a medicinal for respiratory conditions such as bronchitis, asthma and colds. Joseph drinks his powdered lotus root with green tea for his smoking. Andy, a retired vaudevillian, drank lotus tea daily for years to reduce his PSA levels as well as to clear up what he called "the rocks in his head". At 80, Andy with his wife continued to perform benefits in Las Vegas retirement homes until on my birthday in 2004, Andy gave his last performance. True to his profession, Andy left the stage, with a polite bow, a wink of his eye and a wave from his hand as the curtain softly closed to a standing ovation.

Lotus Root Stuffed with Almond

1 Lotus root, washed with ends removed.
2-3 tbsp. almond butter, crunchy or smooth
1 tbsp. white miso.
Spring water.

In a stainless steel pot with a steamer basket:

Steam or pressure cook lotus root until soft but still firm.
Set aside to cool.
Mix miso in warm water until dissolved in a bowl.
Add almond butter to miso.
Mix miso and butter into a paste.
Push almond butter into lotus root through the open ends.
Turn the root in a clock wise manner while filling the Lotus.
When root is full of nut butter, slice.
Serve.

This stuffed lotus root can also be added to soups.

The lotus plant has many medicinal usages. The leaves are used as an astringent for conditions such as diarrhea and sunstroke. The seeds are eaten raw for insomnia, anxiety and as a tonic. The flowers mashed into a powder are made into a tea have been used to treat syphilis and uterine bleeding. The root is used by Japanese Kanpo practitioners for lung disorders, ground into a fine powder and drunk as a tea. I have patients who are smokers and drink lotus tea twice a day to clear their lungs and assist their breathing. The Lotus plant blooms in daylight and closes its petals with the evening to reopen again with the sun. Egyptian mythology associated the lotus plant with rebirth of the soul.

*(**Egyptian Book of the Dead**). Buddhist and Hindu beliefs held the lotus as a fertility symbol. Every aspect of the lotus plant is redeemed for its many medicinal properties as well as inspiration of humanity through faith. Perhaps that is why in **Homer's Odyssey,** Circe, when finding Odysseus and his men, gave them honey and lotus fruit to ease their minds and souls. In Hawaii, lotus root is eaten as a candy by the young, cooked in soups and stews for the infirmed and fried as a tasty appetizer.*

Louise's Stuffed Artichokes

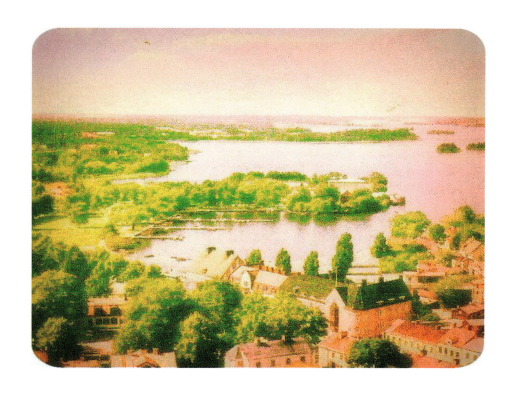

In New Jersey a wonderful patient, Louise, suggested another technique for cooking an artichoke which has proven to be very effective. Struggling with high cholesterol for many years, Louise was quite a champ at the time that I worked with her. She would often say in her best Jersey tone, "I hate your food", gobble down whatever I had prepared and compliment me with a "thank you." Louise runs her household like the captain of a battleship, and is a caregiver to all of her family. A loving woman, a loving wife, and a loving daughter, it is in her honor that I dedicate this version of a stuffed artichoke.

Louise's Stuffed Artichoke

1-3 artichokes, wash, thorns removed.
Olive oil.
Goat/sheep Romano pecorino, sheep/goat feta, crumbled.

Preheat oven to broil:

Wrap artichokes with cooking string in a clockwise manner securing the leaves.

In a stainless steel pot:

Place artichokes in water.
Boil.
Reduce heat.
Simmer for 10-30 minutes until the leaves are soft and tender.
Remove artichokes from pot.

In an oven safe casserole dish:

Place artichokes.
Spread the leaves of the artichoke wide.
Sprinkle olive oil onto the leaves.
Stuff leaves with goat/sheep cheeses.
Broil until cheese is a golden brown.
Serve.

*Artichokes are cultivated in Southern Europe and also in the Northern Mediterranean. Thought to have originated in Northern Africa, artichokes immigrated to Europe and eventually the United States from France and Mexico. Artichokes are a perennial thistle that prefers a warm tropical climate. Traditional preparation of the leaves involved boiling, steaming and frying. The hearts of the artichoke as well as the stem are edible. There are two preferred types of artichokes. The **purple** artichoke is used primarily as a decorative table setting. More familiar is the **green artichoke** which is used in cooking. Tea can be prepared from the artichoke leaves and the extract has been used for constipation Seen in health food stores, artichokes are now used for the lowering of cholesterol. The artichoke in traditional oriental medicine is used to "moisten the lungs" by aiding a dry cough in the form of a tea and also eaten as a food is promoted as a laxative. The plant itself is beautiful when it flowers and will often be grown as a decorative boundary flower in gardens.*

Macro Banana Squash
with Wild Rice

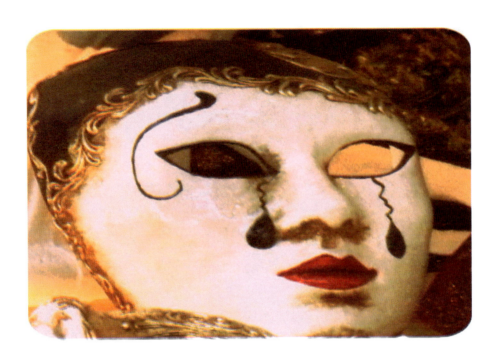

My squash recipe is easy to prepare and a compliment to any meal. One of my patients was a talented textile artist who specialized in mask making. In time he developed **"fibromyalgia"** *in his hands. Cold weather and a damp environment made it almost impossible for him to move his fingers. He was prescribed years of pain medication and combined alcohol to mask his pain. Eventually, it became difficult to separate his dependency to the medications or the pain from his fibromyalgia. His treatment consisted of a full body approach. Addressing the* **"fibromyalgia"** *with his* **substance problems,** *resulted in his complete remission enabling him to return to his craft..*

Macro Banana Squash with Wild Rice

1 banana squash, washed, cut in half lengthwise, de-seeded.2 leeks or green onions, peeled, washed, sliced.
1 cauliflower, broken into florets.
1 cup fresh peas.
2 carrots, sliced.
2-4 tbsp. olive oil.
1 garlic bulb. minced.
1 tbsp. rosemary.
1 tbsp. thyme.
1 cup wild rice, cooked.
° Tsp. black sesame seeds.
Goat/sheep Romano pecorino, feta crumbled

Preheat oven to 350 degrees.

Place a steamer basket into a stainless steel pot.

Place squash, vegetables in basket and pot.
Steam vegetables with banana squash until soft.
Remove from heat.
Remove the meat of the banana squash from the shell.
Place the squash shell aside in an oven safe casserole dish.
Place squash meat in a mixing bowl.
Add in remaining vegetables, rice, herbs and oil.
Place mixture within the shell of banana squash.
Bake at 350 degrees for 30 minutes until a golden brown.
Sprinkle sesame seeds on top.
Sprinkle goat/sheep feta cheese if desired.
Broil for an additional 20 minutes.
Serve.

The Banana squash is a cold winter crop. Originating in Central America , the banana squash migrated to Northern America as *"**seed jewelry**"* in trade from indigenous tribe to indigenous tribe . Similar to their cousin the pumpkin, the banana squash is also rich in vitamins and minerals primarily beta carotene. Cultivated today in India as well as Europe, the banana squash can grow to 2 or more feet in length. Markets in the United States sell the banana squash usually sliced in halves due to their large sizes. Sweet in flavor, the banana squash can be slightly pink to a bright golden yellow in color. A species of banana squash is known as the **Pink Squash**. Native American Indians have traditionally used the banana squash to control parasitical infections by roasting the seeds and consuming them as a tea or food. The uneaten seeds and the rinds were used as a mulch to enrich their soil for planting. Planting the squash was simplistic and direct. Throw the seeds on the ground, push the seeds into the soil, water and walk away.

Macro Primavera Pasta Pie

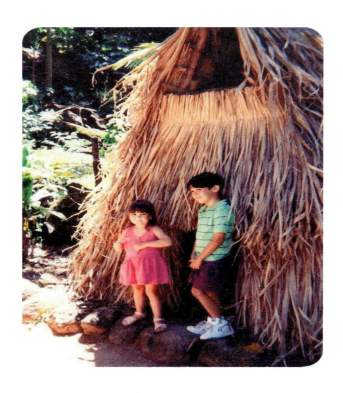

*My **Macro Primavera Pasta Pie** is based on the famous American **"Yankee Doodle Pasta Pie"** from the 1950's. The original Primavera Pie was made from the spaghetti and meatballs left over from the night before. It was mixed, baked and then deep fried until brown and crunchy. Yummy as it was, it caused many a clogged artery while shooting cholesterol levels sky high. In my home there were never any left overs so I always make my Primavera fresh each time. My **Macro Primavera Pasta Pie** is wheat and dairy free, cholesterol friendly and supports the principles of the American Heart Association for a healthy heart.*

Macro Primavera Pasta Pie

Preheat oven to 350 degrees

Crust:

4 oz. spelt spaghetti.
1 cup sheep/goat Romano Pecorino, grated.
2 tbsp. olive oil.

In a stainless steel pot boil water and prepare spaghetti according to package instructions.

Remove from heat.
Drain spaghetti and set aside.
Combine olive oil, cheese.
Stir in spaghetti.
Lightly oil pie pan.
Press spaghetti mixture onto bottom of pie pan.

Set aside.

Filling:

2 tbsp. olive oil.
2 tbsp. garlic powder.
2 cups cauliflower florets.
1 red onion, sliced.
2 cups extra firm tofu, cubed.
1 cup sheep/goat Romano Pecorino, grated.
1 tsp. sweet basil, dry.

In stainless steel skillet:

Heat oil.
Add cauliflower, onion, and tofu.
Cook until the onions are a clear transparency.
Add garlic and spices.
Stir until all ingredients are heated evenly.
Spoon over crust.

Topping:

Goat/sheep feta, crumbled.
1 cup goat/sheep sour cream.
2 tbsp. sheep/goat Romano Pecorino, grated.

Mix feta/sour cream thoroughly in a bowl.
Pour over vegetables filling in pie crust.
Cover.
Bake for 25 minutes.
Uncover.
Sprinkle pecorino over vegetables.
Bake for 10 minutes until browned.
Let stand for 10 minutes.
Serve.

Spelt is believed to have originated in Egypt. As spelt is part of the wheat family, it does produce a small amount of gluten. However, many individuals who are wheat and gluten intolerant can tolerate spelt. Spelt is cultivated throughout Europe and the United States in direct competition with wheat products. Beer and vodka from Poland, flour, pasta, breads and cakes are produced from the spelt grain. The husks of the spelt are used as mulch. Similar in the nutritional values of wheat, many health markets are carrying "spelt grass" sprouted and made into juice or powder as an alternative to wheat grass. The spelt grain produces pale white flour that is fine in quality compared to the brown wheat flour. Spelt is thought to be the original grain from which wheat is cultivated from. Wheat products are derived from wheat berries . Wheat berries are a cold winter crop and have a hard outer shell which can make assimilation and digestion of this grain difficult. Spelt is grown in warm and temperate climate. The husk of the spelt grain is softer than the wheat berry making it easier for digestion as and nutritional assimilation.

My Cabbage Roll Dumplings

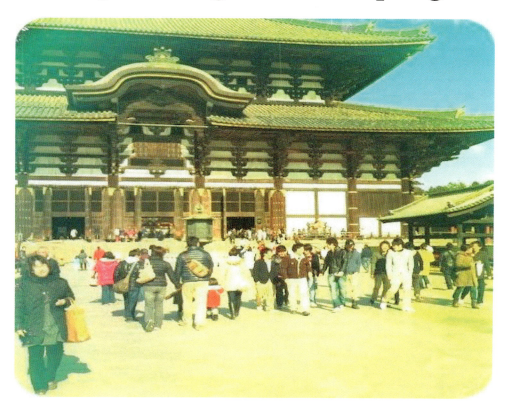

There are many varieties of what is best known as the **"Asian Dumpling"**. *Thailand, Korea, Japan and China all have their country's unique version. The word* **"dumpling"** *is used to describe an assortment of vegetables, fruits, nuts and meats wrapped in pastry flour and then steamed or deep fried. I developed this version of a spring roll for my patient who had cholesterol problems. In celebration of the Chinese New Year spring rolls are made as a pastry dipped in honey and rolled in sugar so as to insure good fortune and prosperity for the year to come.* **My Cabbage Roll** *also inspires good fortune and prosperity*

My Cabbage Roll Dumplings

6 -8 cabbages leafs, washed.
2-3 cups cooked brown rice.
1 leek or red onion sliced, diced.
1 garlic bulb, minced.
Black sesame seeds.
Sesame oil, dark.

In a stainless steel pot:

Steam cabbage.
Put aside.

Sauce:

1 cup corn kernels.
1-2 tbsp. white miso.
Goat/sheep, nondairy milk.
Red, black pepper, chili and saffron to desired taste.

Place fresh corn kernels in a bender/food processor.
Blend until creamy.

In a stainless steel pot:

Combine corn, cheese/yogurt, spices and milk.
Simmer on low for 40-60 minutes.

Set aside.

Cabbage Roll:

In a stainless steel skillet:

Sauté leeks/onions, garlic in oil until the onion is an opaque clear color.
Combine rice, onions, garlic in skillet.
Stir.
Remove from heat.
Place rice mixture in middle of cabbage leafs.
Roll end to end.
Use tooth picks to keep in place at the end of each roll
Cover leafs with sauce and roasted sesame seeds.
Serve.

*Cabbage has many traditional usages as an expeller of parasites, healing ulcers and used topically as a poultice. Often you will see in markets cabbage listed as a "**head cabbage**" which is round and leafy. Head cabbage can have light green, white or purple leaves. I prefer the **Napa Cabbage** otherwise known as **Chinese cabbage** for most of my recipes. Cabbage is very high in Vitamin C and has been used for its anti-inflammatory properties. European midwifes would place a poultice of mashed cabbage on a nursing mothers inflamed breast to relieve the discomfort of engorgement. Today, China is the largest producer of all varieties cabbages followed by India and Russia. Pickled, fermented or made into a beverage, cabbage has a long history as a food source and for medicinal use. The cabbage for many Europeans and Americans was not at first introduced as an eatable food source, but rather as a children's story in the **Adventures of Peter Rabbit by Beatrice Potter**.*

My Colorful Vegetable Casserole

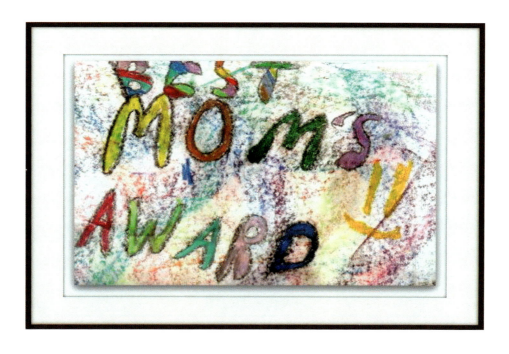

I believe this casserole was invented by harried moms who forgot to go to the market on their way home from their children's soccer, baseball, band and ballet practices while negotiating scout meetings and the **PTA Pot Lucks.** *At least, that was how I arrived at this ancient form of cooking. Whenever I make this casserole dish, I imagine cave moms stirring and throwing into the flames and earthen pots a leg of this and a root of that, all the while instructing their cave children on correct color choices for cave drawing, pulling lice out of their hair, cleaning cave pelts and whatever else cave mom's did in their day. To todays cave mom's, I politely curtsey and say "you go girl".*

My Colorful Vegetable Casserole

Kelp 3-6 inches, washed.
4-6 carrots, sliced.
1 leek/red onion, peeled, washed, sliced.
2-3 zucchini, sliced or 2 cups butternut squash, peeled, quartered, de-seeded.
1 cup string beans, julienne sliced.
1-3 tbsp. olive oil.
½ tsp. each basil, tarragon,
1 garlic bulb, minced.
1 lb. firm tofu, cubed.
1 lb. sheep/goat feta marinated in olive oil/ minced garlic.

Preheat oven to 350 degrees.

Lightly oil kelp by dipping in a bowl of olive oil.
Wipe excessive oil from the kelp with a paper towel.

Place kelp on bottom of oven safe casserole dish.
Layer carrots on top of kelp.
Sprinkle with garlic, basil, tarragon, olive oil.
Layer squash on top.
Sprinkle with dry herbs.
Layer onions on top.
Sprinkle with herbs.
Layer feta or tofu or both over vegetables, herbs, oil.
Bake covered for 1 hour.
Remove lid
Bake for 15 minutes.
Broil until feta/tofu is a golden brown.
Serve.

*The word "**casserole**" has two literal meanings with in the Webster dictionary. One literally meaning: "**a recipe that combines food and is slowly cooked**," while the other meaning defines the "**cookware, dish, or pot**" in use. The origin of the casserole is believed to have originated in Greece and then moved throughout European and Asian rural kitchens until English royalty developed a desire for what was originally a type of "**Shepherd's pie**". The casserole was brought over to the North Americas as a result for the need of a hearty meal that could be prepared quickly. The word "**casserole**," is French for a "**bowl to cook in**". Today the word "**casserole**" has many meanings. The original casserole recipe incorporated rice shaped into the form of a pot or dish and then filled with meats, vegetables and grains. Today, the most famous American casserole dish is the "**tuna casserole**," and "**macaroni and cheese**" next to mine, of course.*

My Own Escarole Soup

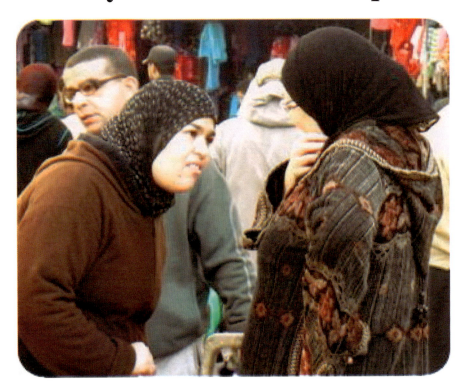

*Traveling throughout Europe I had the opportunity to taste many different foods. While in Casablanca I became lost in the **casbar** looking for "**Rick's Place**". Unable to locate Humphrey Bogart or Ingrid Bergman, I did find streets and alleyways of market vendors. Casablanca is primarily a Middle Eastern community dominated by men who manage the markets and would not speak to me or allow any photographs. This recipe came from behind the market stands where the women prepared the meals to sale. Language is not a necessity when cooking. Love for the passion of the food and the desire this passion evokes is a language all by itself.*

My Own Escarole Soup

1 head of escarole, rinsed.
½ cup wakame, washed.
1 6-8 inch ginger root, minced
4 cups of water.
1-2 tbsp. white miso.
1 leek or green onion, peeled, sliced.
Olive oil.

In a stainless steel pot:

Boil water.
Reduce heat to simmer.
Add escarole and ginger.
Simmer for 30 minutes.
Reduce to low.

In stainless steel skillet:

Sauté leeks in oil.
Add to pot.
Add wakame and miso to pot.
Simmer for 15 minutes until miso is dissolved.
Serve.

Escarole is a bitter, broad leaf winter vegetable that belongs in the daisy family of botanicals. Listed as an endive, the escarole has hearty leaves that can be steamed, boiled in a soup or eaten raw as a salad. Escarole has a slightly bitter flavor. When cooked in a soup this bitterness is not as strong as it is when eaten raw. Traditional practitioners of oriental medicine believe that bitter flavors influence and aid the smooth flow of the liver and gall bladder breakdown of food. This could be interpreted today with standard medical evaluation of the escarole's peristaltic effect upon the body. The function of the liver with the gall bladder play an important role in the production of "bile" which aids the body in production of gastric acids that influence digestion and assist in the breakdown of food. Escarole has traditional usage for constipation due to the high concentration of magnesium and as a plant fiber. Relatively new to the American plate, escarole is finding its way into many kitchens as a healthy way to include another leafy green vegetable into the diet.

Nana's Sugar Peas

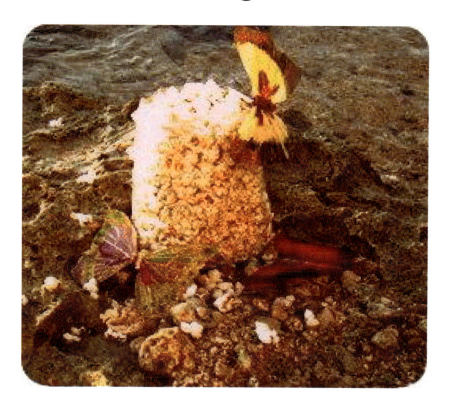

*My auntie passed away on Memorial Day, 2003 at St. Rose Hospital in Las Vegas, Nevada. Her favorite food at 82 was overly buttered theater popcorn. As well as giving my auntie her popcorn, I also prepared for her this recipe. Often she would say, "I prefer white rice not this brown rice and it needs more salt". On my way home from treating a small boy in the New Mexico desert, I received a message from St. Rose Hospital that she had relapsed. As I spoke to her on the phone, before she closed her eyes, she said **"I will be waiting for you and bring my popcorn"**. I hope this holds her over until I see her again. Aloha.*

Nana's Sugar Peas

4 cups sugar peas.
1-3 tbsp. virgin olive oil.
1 tsp. garlic powder.
1 cup almond, slivered.

Preheat oven to 450 degrees.

Spread sugar peas in an oven safe baking dish.
Sprinkle with olive oil/garlic.
Roast for 10 minutes.
Remove from oven.
Spread almonds evenly over the top.
Return to oven.
Bake until almonds are slightly brown.
Serve over brown rice.

Sugar peas or snow peas are from the family of the green pea. Sugar peas can be eaten whole including the pod. Originating from Asia, these peas will grow at the end of spring and be ready for harvest at the beginning of winter. They are cold weather crops and often used in Oriental cooking. Grown both on vines or close to the ground sugar peas are very delicate and their cultivation is the most difficult to maintain of all the pea family. Subject to plights from insects, weather, and animals often hinder the harvest of the sugar pea increasing the cost for production. High in magnesium and other vitamins, sugar peas provide an excellent food choice with hypertensive diets. Commercial use as ingredients in pet foods and garden mulch. By far the sweetest of all legumes within the pea family, the sugar pea provides the best of all choices for a fresh ingredient in salads and in Asian cooking is the most sought after vegetable in stir fries, soups and sauces.

Popeyed Spinach Turnovers

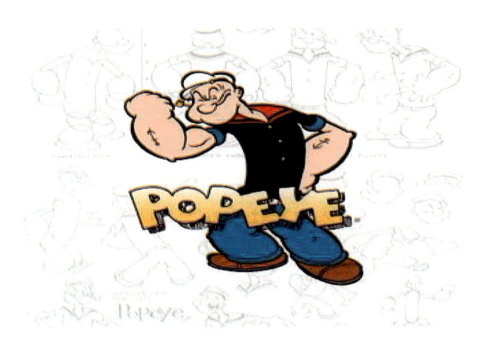

In 1984, I was asked to treat the retired Ambassador to Jamaica's cook in San Francisco. The house was three stories high, the rooms decorated in black and gold. The cook was a wonderful woman from Germany who suffered from coronary heart disease. We sat in the kitchen for hours comparing recipes. I suggested for her to cease all cow products and replace them with goat or sheep. Goat and sheep products have less concentrated fats and oils making it easier to digest. So, we made **Popeyed Spinach Turnovers** together for a *"fabulous party for the rich and famous"*. While cooking, a Rockefeller popped his head in and attempted a pre party appetizer. We quickly waved him away and locked the kitchen door.

Popeyed Spinach Turnovers

Preheat oven to 350 degrees:

1 onion, chopped.
2 lb. fresh spinach, chopped.
1 lb. zucchini, sliced.
1 lb. extra firm, cubed.
1 cup wakame broken into pieces
½ cup fine dry bread wheat/yeast free crumbs
Non Dairy sour cream.
1 cup sheep/ goat Romano Pecorino, grated.
4 tbsp. olive oil.
½ teaspoon each pepper, basil, oregano.
Goat/Sheep feta marinade (See below)

Preheat oven to 350 degrees.

In a stainless steel skillet:

Sauté spinach, onion, wakame, zucchini in olive oil until onions are a clear opaque.
Remove from heat.

In a bowl.

Mash tofu into fine pieces.
Add cheeses.
Stir in spinach/vegetable mixture to tofu/cheese.
Place in a well-oiled oven safe casserole dish.
Sprinkle 2 tbsp. pecorino on spinach.
Bake uncovered for 35 minutes, or until edges begin to brown.
Top spinach with marinated

Feta marinade:

Marinate feta in 2-4 tbsp. (or more) of olive oil.
Fold in fresh rosemary minced garlic.
Blend.
Refrigerate for a few hours to soften the rosemary.
The longer the marinate ages the stronger the taste.
Broil until golden brown.
Serve.

*Spinach is a dark leafy green vegetable that began its history iIndia and was given as a gift by the king of Nepal to China. From Asia, spinach made its way to Europe via Persian Moors. Spinach is still one of the most disliked vegetables (**Wikipedia**, **the free encyclopedia**) in the world. Very high in iron and calcium as well as other minerals and vitamins, spinach is an excellent vegetable choice. During the late 1930's, food rationing had begun to take effect all throughout Europe. A declining economy and the advent of war produced a shortage in all production of commerce creating a worldwide food shortage. The few vegetables that were available were sent overseas to these starving populations by the United States. The one vegetable that remained in abundance was spinach. As the most disliked vegetable at that time it was necessary to incorporate media to increase spinach consumption. As a war effort, **POPEYE** was created to symbolize strength and hope which was restored to him when he ate spinach that was usually given to him by his girlfriend, **OLIVE OIL.** To this day when I use spinach I always include OLIVE Oil, because*
"I am what I am".

Sauté Almond French Long Green Beans

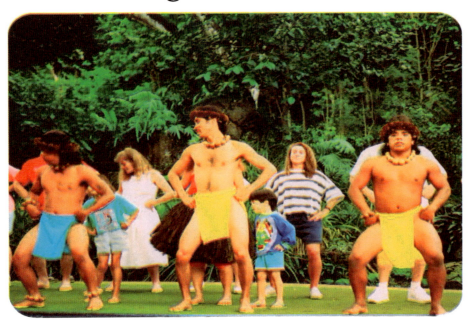

On Christmas Day of 2003, I had my Annual Christmas Party and 5 pounds of **Sauté Almond French Long Green Beans**. *In the traditional, "oh my bananas, I forgot this and that" and "who else is coming" and the ever popular, " of course you can bring them" resulted in my pajama flight to the local market. Returning home, my children, most particularly my banchi son, were all over the place with friends and Christmas toys. Then I saw the kitchen void of most of the Christmas feast, specifically, the* **Sauté Almond French Long Green Beans.** *I quickly recovered the feast but to this day my children can still recite at length when mom went* **"French"** *over her beans.*

Sauté Almond French Long Green Beans

1 lb. long green beans, washed, ends cut.
4-6 carrots, sliced
1 leek or green onions, peeled, washed, sliced.
3 bulbs garlic, minced.
1 tbsp. sweet basil.
2-4 tbsp. olive oil.
Garlic powder to taste.
Goat/sheep feta marinated in olive oil.
Sliced toasted almonds.

Preheat oven to 350 degrees.

In an oven safe casserole dish:

Arrange a layer of carrots evenly on the bottom.
Sprinkle oil over carrots.
Layer with garlic powder then onions then green beans then garlic bulbs
Repeat layering until all ingredients are gone.
Bake at 350 degrees uncovered for 1 hour.
Remove from oven.
Sprinkle with almonds, feta.
Broil until almonds and feta are brown.
Serve over brown rice, millet, etc.

*Green beans belong to the Fabaceae family of legumes. The "green bean" refers to the beans within the pods which are young and unripe. The green bean is a vine that will grow with the assistance of a trestle. The bean attached to a trestle can grow up to 12 feet in height or more. The tallest green bean and the most famous green bean reported is the one that Jack climbed in the European folk story, "**Jack and the Beanstalk**" where a bean splits in two and sprouts up to a giant's castle. Green beans are very high in magnesium and plant fiber. The green been is loaded with the antioxidants Vitamin C, A and E as well as digestible protein. A unique legume, the green bean is easy to cultivate and has many commercial uses. As an added ingredient for pet foods, mulch for horticulture as well as a food source for human consumption. Traditional oriental practitioners include green beans in many food based formulas for cardiovascular conditions, hypertension and cholesterol. Green beans are also be effective due to the chlorophyll as an excellent choice as a plant fiber for constipation.*

Snuffy's Peas Pilaf

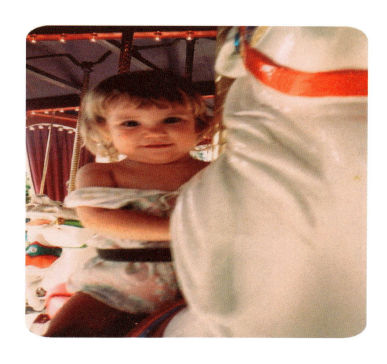

My first experience with "peas" was when I fled to an emergency room in California with my daughter. At 15 months she was "snuffing". This meant that she was trying her hardest to sneeze something out of her nose. I had no idea what was wrong except that she was frantic which made me frantic. The emergency room doctor suggested surgery. I looked at the nurse, the nurse looked at me and we turned my daughter upside down. Looking up into her nostrils we found many petite green peas. Gently rinsing out the peas from her little nose, I carried Alicia home. Needless to say, peas are not my favorite legume, though they are my daughter's who eats them regularly without placing them in her nose.

Snuffy's Peas Pilaf

2 cups cooked brown rice.
1 cup fresh garden peas, shelled.
2 tbsp. olive oil.
1 leek or green onion, peeled, washed, sliced.
3-4 tbsp. raw cashews, chopped.
2-3 tbsp. golden currents.
1 Cinnamon stick.
1 bay leaf.
3 peppercorns.

In a stainless steel pan:

Sauté peas, leek/onions, cashews, currants in olive oil until tender.
Add bay leaf, cinnamon and peppercorns.
Toss ingredients together.
Remove from heat.
Serve over cooked brown rice

Peas are fresh legumes removed from their pods. Grown on vines above the ground, peas are cool weather crops. There are many varieties of peas. This recipe calls for fresh garden peas that have already been removed from their shells. Peas can be dried and stored as a hard legume for later use. Cooked into soups, stews or ground into flour, peas are a good choice as a vegetable protein and are found in many cultures. Asian practitioners of traditional oriental medicine use a species of peas as a tonic in some of the food source formulas to regain strength. Commercial use of peas includes pet foods, vitamin supplements as well as an ingredient in green drinks. Peas are a staple part of many meals. The most famous food combinations are: carrots and peas, pea soup and peas in a pod. Americans worldwide still embrace the 1930's cartoon character "Sweet Pea" of Popeye fame which for many a parent was their children's first introduction to peas. From media to the mouths of babes, parent to parent anything that works in having our children try new foods that are good for them is most appreciated.

Stuffed Kabocha Squash

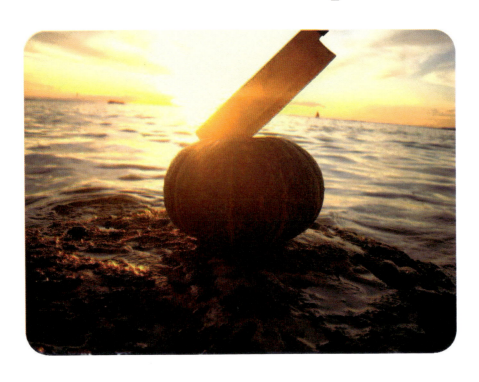

My patients really love this recipe. However, some experience great difficulty when cutting through the tough rind of the Japanese Kabocha squash. I had a patient who was a medical doctor from Great Britain. He was diagnosed with "Parkinson like" symptoms for over twenty years. In one treatment his tremors of the upper limbs ceased and his condition improved daily. He is now in retirement with his wife who does most of the cooking. Oh yes, for the slicing of the pumpkin. Take a very sharp heavy cleaver. Place paper towels on the counter and slam the cleaver into the rind. Then with a strong heavy heave, slam it against the counter. Usually it will break in half. If not, try the floor.

Stuffed Kabocha Squash

1 kabocha squash cut in half and de-seeded.
1 ½ cup cauliflower florets.
4-6 carrots, sliced.
1-2 leeks or green onions, sliced.
1 garlic bulb, minced.
1 tsp. sweet basil.
Goat/sheep Pecorino Romano, grated.
Goat/sheep, feta crumbled.
2 cups cooked millet.

Preheat oven to 350 degrees.

In a stainless steel pot with a steamer basket:

Steam squash, carrots, cauliflower until soft but firm.
Drain water and remove vegetables from pot.
Scoop out the meat of the squash from its shell.
Place kabocha and vegetables in mixing bowl.
Save the shell.
Set aside.

In a stainless steel skillet:

Sauté garlic, leeks/onion in olive oil.
Mix cauliflower, carrots, leeks/onions, spices, kabocha together.
Combine millet to vegetable mixture.
Place mixture in the kabocha shell.
Sprinkle cheeses on top.
Bake at 350 for 15-20 minutes.
Broil till brown.
Serve

Kabocha squash is a Japanese pumpkin similar to the American pumpkin with a very strong rind. Orange to bright yellow depending on the grower, the meat of the kabocha is very sweet in comparison to other gourds. Composed of antioxidants, minerals and vitamins, the kabocha squash when combined with the ingredients in this recipe creates a balanced meal. The seeds of the kabocha can be roasted and salted for their anti-parasitical properties. The squash can be stuffed, mashed, fried into patties or pureed into a soup. The kabocha is very high in the beta carotene which is very beneficial for the healing and repair of the skin. As an antioxidant, beta-carotene is also useful for digestive disorders such as constipation. The kabocha can also be grated into a salad and eaten raw. The kabocha as a vegetable is very high in digestible plant fiber. This makes the kabocha a desirable vegetable to combine with a grain creating a complete nutritional profile. The grain millet is used in this recipe to enhance easy assimilation for protein, minerals and B vitamins.

STUFFED SWEET MAUI ONIONS

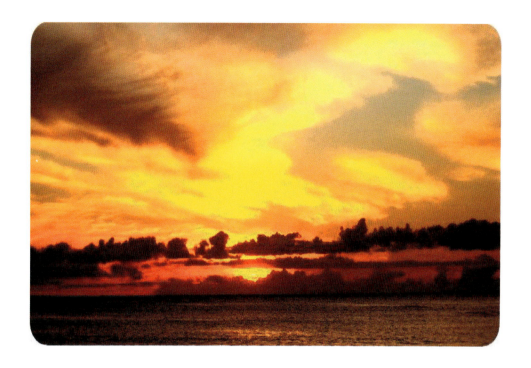

My patient was a thirty year retired Air Force Lt. Colonel and a retired pilot for American Airlines. He was referred after his microwave treatments resulted in elevated PSA levels and a enlarged the prostrate. He also had elevated cholesterol, thyroid and platelet problems. After 10 days of treatment, his PSA levels dropped within an acceptable range and his other conditions improved. Returning home to Las Vegas, Nevada, he and his wife once a year return to Honolulu to play golf, see me, and to eat their **"Stuffed Sweet Maui Onions.**

STUFFED SWEET MAUI ONIONS

6 Maui or sweet yellow onions, skin peeled, washed.
1 ½ cup cooked millet or brown rice.
Steamed veggies (carrots, squash. cauliflower, etc.)
2 cloves garlic, minced.
Olive oil/olive oil sprays to taste.
Goat/sheep feta or sheep Romano pecorino, grated.

Preheat oven to 350 degrees.

In a stainless steel pot place a steamer basket:

Steam onions until soft but firm 10-20 minutes.

Remove the core of the onions leaving only the shells (this can be done by using a **sharp paring knife and cut clockwise around the last ring of the onion which will loosen the outside of the onion** and then with the tip of the knife or a fork pierce the middle and remove the center).
The remaining pulp can be frozen and added to soups, spreads, etc.

In a bowl:

Mix grains with vegetables.

In an oven safe casserole dish:

Stuff vegetables/grains within the onions and top with the feta, pecorino or both.
Bake at 350 degrees for 15 minutes.
Broil till top is a golden brown
Garnish with parsley or a lemon wedge.
Serve.

Traditional usages for the onion family have been many. Folk remedies for onions are used to improve breathing, as an anti-parasitical, for warts, to grow hair and to eliminate hair. Onions are essential in Indian and Chinese cooking. Garlic is viewed as a hot herb in Chinese medicinal formulas. Onions are considered to be somewhat cooler in a food based formula and easier to assimilate. Egyptian Pharaohs were traditionally buried with wreaths of onions which symbolized the birth/death/rebirth cycle for eternal life. It was also believed that the vapors from the onion would revive the dead if not in this life then in the next **(Egyptian Book of the Dead)**. *High in antioxidants, onions are believed to enhance the body's immune system in conditions such as osteoporosis, diabetes, and infertility. Onion tea, poultices of mashed onion, onions rubbed over sore muscles, onion oil in the ear for an ear ache, onion wine, onion brandy, and onions for sunstroke are just a few of the folk remedies still referred to today. Onions like their relative the garlic have a high concentration of sulfur within their peel. This may be why onions are so odorous though healthy.*

Wok a Tok

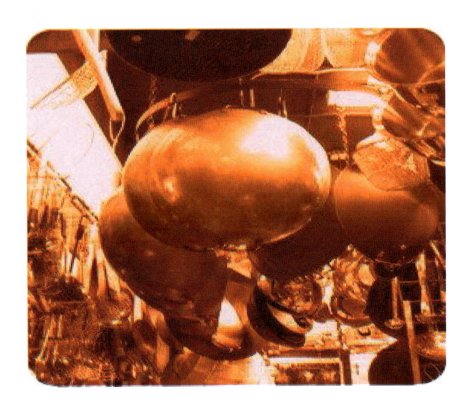

Everyone in Hawaii cooks with a wok. It was not until I returned to the U.S. mainland that I realized that woks are not very popular outside of Asian communities. Cooking for the first few times on the East Coast was challenging. Whether I was in Maryland, New Jersey, or New York, no one had any idea what a **stainless steel non electric Teflon free carbonized wok** *was or where I could purchase one. My very industrious patient, David, located my first East Coast wok somewhere in New Jersey. Ten years later, David still has the wok and cooks at home with it whenever he has the urge for my* **"Wok a talk"** *recipe.*

Wok a Tok

1 cauliflower, broken into florets.
Carrots, sliced.
Chinese cabbage, sliced, quartered.
Onions or leeks, peeled, washed, sliced.
1 cup snow peas.
1 zucchini, cut into half-moons.
1 lb. firm tofu, cubed.
1 cup bean sprouts.
Wakame seaweed rinsed, soaked in water until soft.
1 garlic bulb, minced.
4-6 inch ginger root, grated.
2-3 olive oil.
Braggs Amino Acids or wheat free tamari.

In a bowl:

Marinade tofu in Braggs/tamari with ginger.
Set aside.

In stainless steel skillet/wok.

Heat oil.
Stir onions, leeks, garlic, carrots, and cauliflower into the skillet/wok using a wooden spatula.
Drain tofu, wakame from bowl.
Dry with a paper towel.
Place all ingredients in wok/skillet.
Add root vegetables, cabbage, zucchini, and snow peas. bean sprouts.
Stir and toss quickly until all vegetables are evenly cooked.
Serve over rice

Woks are traditional skillets found throughout Asia. The wok's raised edges or "lips" allow for cooking with small amounts of oil in preparation of the many dishes that require stir frying. The oil can be moved around the sides of the wok by rotating the wok and quickly moving the ingredients with a spatula. Traditional woks were made of cast iron and carbonized steel. Woks were originally designed to be used over a pit stove where the heat rising from the flames was fully directed at the bottom of the wok. The wok would typically sit in these wooden or coal based stoves within the stove top, sunk within the flame to insure even cooking. Today in Oriental restaurants pit stoves are powered by natural gas with the burners recessed below the stove's surface. Though not as useful as the pit stoves, modern households with their flat ranges can remove their burner cover and place a wok ring for the wok to sit on for a more traditional style of cooking. Woks are in use today primarily in Asia and Japan. Steel based woks are still mainly in use in these countries. Teflon coated f woks for easier cleaning and electric style range woks are quickly replacing the traditional.

American Macro Sweet Potato Pie

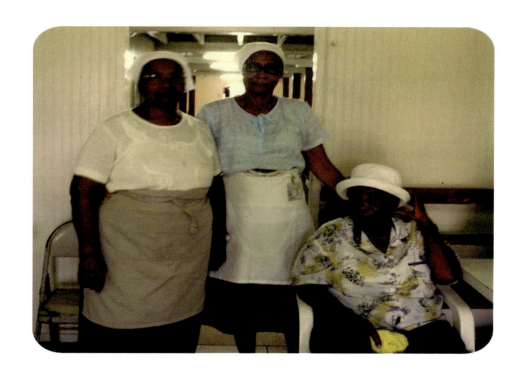

*A 16th century European food, **Sweet Potato Pie** was widely regarded as an aphrodisiac and enjoyed by members of the royal court. Very similar to yams, the sweet potato was eventually incorporated into cultural foods. Eventually the Sweet potato pie made its way to the Americas and has become recognized with African Americans as "**Soul Food**.". The crust for this **Sweet Potato Pie** can be interchanged with an amaranth crust or other wheat free crusts. Extra cinnamon also enhances the flavor of the sweet potato as does letting the mixture sit overnight prior to baking. Thank you ladies from the **Angelina Church in Antigua** for this recipe.*

American Macro Sweet Potato Pie

2-3 cups of Sweet potato steamed, de-seeded, cut into quarters.
1-2 lbs. tofu cream cheese or nondairy cream cheese.
2 8 oz. hazelnut or almond amasake.
1 tbsp. non-alcohol vanilla or almond extract.
1 tsp. pumpkin pie spice.
1 tsp. cinnamon.
½ ground ginger.
Sliced almonds or hazelnuts.
1 cup sucanat, honey, or sweet brown rice syrup, agave.

Blend potato meat in a food processor/blender.
Add in cream cheese, amasake, spices and sweeteners.
Blend.
Place in 9"wheat free pie crust (see below for recipe).
Garnish with nuts.

Crust:

1 cup Amaranth grain.
1 cup soy, goat, or sweet butter, soften or olive oil.
Sliced hazelnuts or almonds.

In stainless steel pot:

Boil water.
Add amaranth.
Reduce heat.
Simmer for 15-20 minutes until the water has evaporated.

Cover pot.

Remove from burner.

Let cool about 5 to 10 minutes.
Mix butter or oil in with amaranth.

Press amaranth mixture into pie pan.

Add kabocha filling.
Top with nuts if desired (hazelnuts for hazelnut amasake, almonds for almond amasake).

Refrigerate 2-4 hours or overnight before eating.
Or
Bake at 350 degrees in the oven for 30-40 minutes until firm.
Serve.

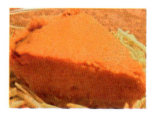

Christmas Rice Pudding

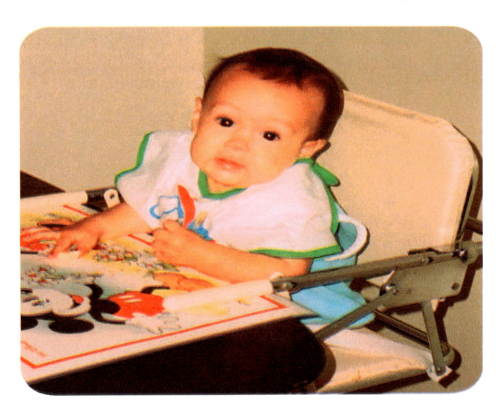

Many of my patients are parents with young children. By the time these families had arrived at my clinic, they had consumed years of medication, artificial colored microwaved foods and pounds of Halloween candy . Rashes, allergies, juvenile onset diabetes and childhood obesity were not unusual in my clinic. In treating families and helping them with their food choices, I realized that I had to create recipes that everyone felt comfortable with and would eat. **Christmas Rice Pudding** *is my version of a traditional recipe. This is a favorite in my family and I hope in yours.*

Christmas Rice Pudding

1-2 cups cooked brown rice.
4 cups vanilla soy, rice, almond or goat milk.
Cinnamon to taste.

There are 2 ways to prepare this recipe:

Stove top:

In a stainless steel pot:

Place cooked rice
Add enough milk to cover the rice with an additional inch or more.
Heat on low until milk slightly bubbles.
Remove immediately from heat.
Sprinkle liberally with cinnamon.
Or
Preheat oven to 350 degrees.

Mix milk with cooked rice to desired thickness.
Place mixture in oven safe casserole dish.
Bake for 30-45 minutes.
Sprinkle cinnamon to taste.
Serve.

As an added treat, blue berries, dates etc.
can be stirred in or sprinkled

Rice was first cultivated in Asia and is one of the oldest grains in the world. California is one of the world largest producers of rice today. There are many cultivated varieties of rice. Red rice, wild rice, forbidden rice, Thai, sushi, basmati, and jasmine. Long rice, short rice, sweet rice and black rice compose only a few of the many still to be named varieties of rice. The original rice was a brown rice which is white rice with the husks of the grain still attached and traditionally was eaten only by the poorest of the population Nurturing warming and building in nature; rice can be prepared in many ways. In the Middle East, rice as a pudding is made with white rice flour, where as in India, rice cooked into a pudding will use the whole rice grain and often will include pistachios and raw sugar as ingredients. The use of goat milk for the making of rice pudding was used in Roman times as a "tonic" to build strength. Throughout the world, rice pudding has found its way into households in one form or another. A thin "gruel" for stomach aches, a thicker "rice porridge" for the infirmed and convalescing and "rice pudding" as a beautiful Christmas dessert.

Holiday Kabocha Pumpkin Pie

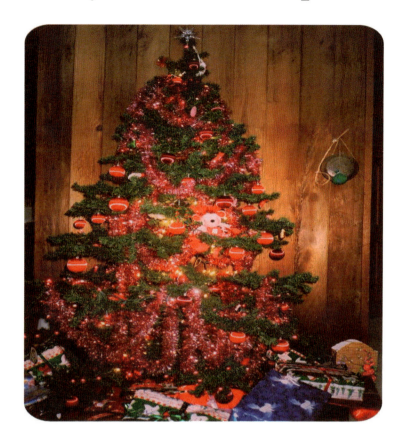

The meat of the kabocha squash is much sweeter than its cousin the pumpkin and a good alternative when making the **traditional pumpkin pie**. *Native to Asia, the kabacha is a newcomer to American and European supermarkets. Its texture and flavor blends well in any recipe where a pumpkin is used whether it is a butternut, acorn or banana. As the kabocha is very sweet, when using the meat to make pies, less added sweeteners are used making this a " sugar friendly" recipe. Each year, I ask my family what they would like me to prepare for Christmas and* **Holiday Kabocha Pumpkin Pie** *is at the top of the list.*

Holiday Kabocha Pumpkin pie

2-3 cups of Kabocha steamed, de-seeded, cut into quarters.
1-2 lbs. tofu cream cheese or nondairy cream cheese.
2 8 oz. hazelnut or almond amasake.
1 tbsp. non-alcohol vanilla or almond extract.
1 tsp. pumpkin pie spice.
1 tsp. cinnamon.
Half teaspoon ground ginger.
Sliced almonds or hazelnuts.
1 cup sucanat, honey, sweet brown rice syrup or agave.

Blend squash meat in a food processor/ blender till smooth.
Add in cream cheese, amasake, spices and sweeteners.
Blend.

Place in 9"wheat free pie crust. (see below for one type of crust).
Garnish with nuts.

Crust:

1 cup Amaranth grain.
1 cup soy, goat or sweet butter, soften or olive oil.
Sliced hazelnuts or almonds.

In stainless steel pot:

Boil water.
Add amaranth.
Reduce heat.
Simmer for 15-20 minutes until the water has evaporated.

170

Cover pot.

Remove from burner.

Let cool about 5 to 10 minutes.
Mix butter or oil in with amaranth

Press amaranth mixture into pie pan.

Add kabocha filling.
Top with nuts if desired. (hazelnuts for hazelnut amasake, almonds for almond amasake).

Refrigerate 2-4 hours or overnight before eating.
Or
Bake at 350 degrees in the oven for 30 degrees for 30-40 minutes until firm.
Serve

Letting this pie sit for a few hours or refrigerating the pie overnight will deepen the taste of this very special Holiday pie, while baking lends a more traditional feel with the aroma of cinnamon and nutmeg wafting throughout the house

*The kabocha squash, a Japanese pumpkin, is related closely to the orange American pumpkin. The Kabocha's rind is of a thinner texture than the American pumpkin and the meat of the kabocha is richer in taste. Loaded with antioxidants, vitamins, and minerals the Kabocha squash is a staple in Japanese households. The seeds when dried and roasted are eaten traditionally as an anti-parasitical and given for constipation. The Kabocha squash combines well with the Central American grain, "**amaranth**". Amaranth is a unique grain that has been in use for over 8000 years. Amaranth was used by the Incas' and Aztecs' culture to build endurance. Amaranth consists of 30 % more digestible protein than rice, wheat, oats and rye. Amaranth can be made into flour, boiled, steamed and mashed into a poultice. Amaranth has been used in folk medicine for hypertension, diabetes, cardiovascular disease and to lower cholesterol. A very sustainable crop, amaranth was rediscovered in the 1970's in the Americas and Mexico as an "energy food" and is manufactured for cereals and included in energy bars as a breakfast food.*

ALOHA

and

Mahalo

Alicia

Alexander

and

Mom

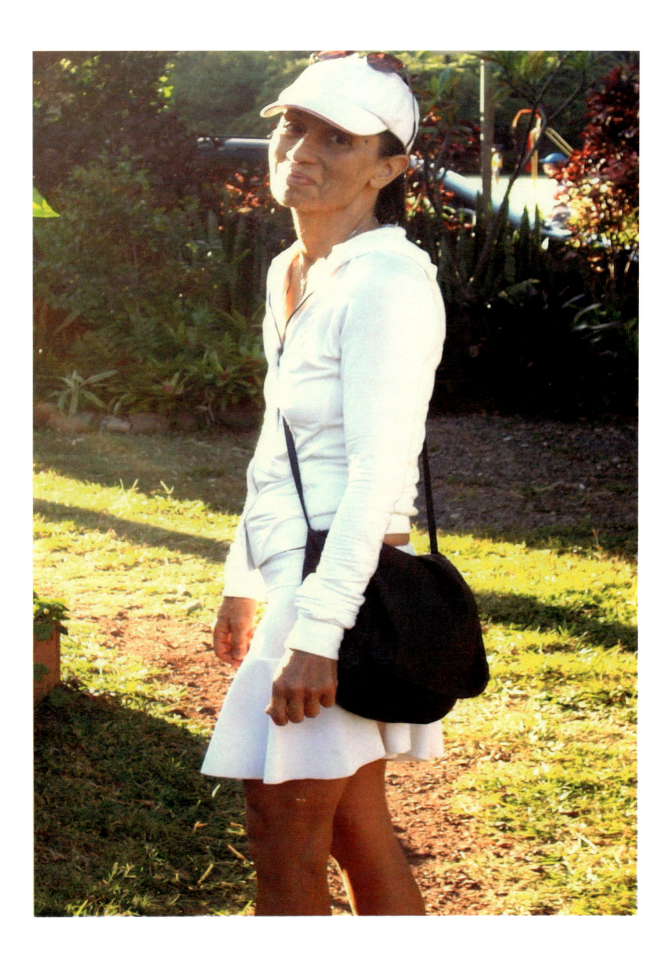

Glossary

Amaranth High in protein and the amino acid lysine, it is a popular grain in Latin American and certain parts of Africa.

Amasake A fermented sweet rice drink often the base for deserts and custards.

Arame A large leaf sea vegetable under the category of sea weeds A shorter cooking time and an excellent source of calcium, and protein.

Arrowroot Japanese "cornstarch" used for thickening soups, etc.

Azuki Beans A small red bean cultivated in Japan. High in potassium and protein.

Barley A cold weather grain similar to rye and wheat.

Cannellini Native to Italy, this is a creamy white bean high very in protein.

Chervil An aromatic herb similar to tarragon.

Chickpeas Also known as "garbanzo beans". Familiar in many Middle Eastern countries.

Cornmeal Traditional Italians are familiar with this grain as "polenta" a coarsely ground corn meal.

Daikon   A Japanese white radish used to aide in digestion of oils and fats.

Flax Seeds   Rich in omegas 3 ,6, and 9.   Flax seeds are best ground and sprinkled at room temperature on salads, soups and vegetables.
Often flax seeds are cold pressed into oils for a more concentrated form of omegas.

Hiziki   In the family of sea vegetables , this sea weed is reported to benefit the growth of hair in Japanese folk medicine.

Horseradish   A member of the mustard family, this root vegetable is hot and spicy often used with oily meals for digestion.

Kombu   A sea vegetable known as "kelp", has been used commercially for its nutritional values.

Legumes   A botanical family including beans, lentils, peanuts and peas.

Lentils   A small variety of beans that has been cultivated throughout the world.   Used for its high protein content

Millet   The "Golden Grain" millet is native to Asia, and was given at one time in China only to pregnant or lactating women. Very high in digestible protein.

Miso   A fermented paste made from soybeans, brown, white, sweet rice or barley. Traditionally used to strengthen   the body miso is convelesance.

Mochi	Mochi is made by cooking sweet brown rice into a glutinous ball then pounding it into a a thin square and baking it until crispy. Traditionally used when traveling long distances and eaten to increase strength and stamina.
Mung beans	Used mostly in sprouted form.
Nori	Japanese seaweed origanlly a paste made into a thin edible sheet in the Edo period through the art of paper making.
Quinoa	Small soft grain native to the Andes.
Rice milk	A vegan drink produced from white or brown rice.
Soba	Noodles that are made from buckwheat or yam flour. A staple in Japan.
Tamari **(soysauce).**	A fermented sauce that results with the making of miso. Heavier in taste than the traditional shoyu
Toasted **sesame oil**	An oil extracted from toasted sesames.
Tofu	Derived from soybeans high in protein made by extracting the curd of coagulated soymilk then pressing it into bricks (squares).
Udon	Flat noodles traditionally made from wheat, also made from buckwheat and brown rice flour.

Ume plums	The alkazelser of Japan. Made from small green plums then pickled for at least one year. Also known as the umeboshi plums these plums are very alkalizing to the body.
Wakame	The most delicate of the kelp family. Wakame requires only be washed and soaked in preparation for eating
Wasabi	A root vegetable similar to horse radish.

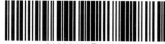

Made in the USA
Lexington, KY
03 March 2013